Also Available From the American Academy of Pediatrics

Common Conditions

ADHD: What Every Parent Needs to Know

Allergies and Asthma: What Every Parent Needs to Know

My Child Is Sick! Expert Advice for Managing Common Illnesses and Injuries

Waking Up Dry: A Guide to Help Children Overcome Bedwetting

Developmental, Behavioral, and Psychosocial Information

CyberSafe: Protecting and Empowering Kids in the Digital World of Texting, Gaming, and Social Media

Mental Health, Naturally: The Family Guide to Holistic Care for a Healthy Mind and Body

The Wonder Years: Helping Your Baby and Young Child Successfully Negotiate the Major Developmental Milestones

Immunization Information

Immunizations & Infectious Diseases: An Informed Parent's Guide

Newborns, Infants, and Toddlers

Baby & Child Health: The Essential Guide From Birth to 11 Years

Caring for Your Baby and Young Child: Birth to Age 5*

Dad to Dad: Parenting Like a Pro

Guide to Toilet Training*

Heading Home With Your Newborn: From Birth to Reality

Mommy Calls: Dr. Tanya Answers Parents' Top 101 Questions About Babies and Toddlers

New Mother's Guide to Breastfeeding*

Newborn Intensive Care: What Every Parent Needs to Know

Raising Twins: From Pregnancy to Preschool

Your Baby's First Year*

Nutrition and Fitness

Food Fights: Winning the Nutritional Challenges of Parenthood Armed With Insight, Humor, and a Bottle of Ketchup

A Parent's Guide to Childhood Obesity: A Road Map to Health

Nutrition: What Every Parent Needs to Know

Sports Success R_x! Your Child's Prescription for the Best Experience

School-aged Children and Adolescents

Building Resilience in Children and Teens: Giving Kids Roots and Wings

Caring for Your School-Age Child: Ages 5 to 12

Caring for Your Teenager

Less Stress, More Success: A New Approach to Guiding Your Teen Through College Admissions and Beyond

For more information, please visit the official AAP Web site for parents, www.HealthyChildren.org/bookstore.

*This book is also available in Spanish.

AUTISM
SPECTRUM DISORDERS

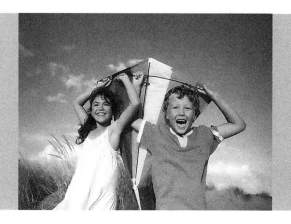

What Every Parent Needs to Know

EDITORS

ALAN I. ROSENBLATT, MD, FAAP

PAUL S. CARBONE, MD, FAAP

WITH WINNIE YU

American Academy of Pediatrics

DEDICATED TO THE HEALTH OF ALL CHILDREN™

American Academy of Pediatrics Department of Marketing and Publications Staff

Director, Department of Marketing and Publications
Maureen DeRosa, MPA

Director, Division of Product Development
Mark Grimes

Manager, Consumer Publishing
Carolyn Kolbaba

Coordinator, Product Development
Holly Kaminski

Director, Division of Publishing and Production Services
Sandi King, MS

Editorial Specialist
Jason Crase

Print Production Specialist
Shannan Martin

Manager, Graphic Design and Production
Peg Mulcahy

Manager, Consumer Marketing and Sales
Kathleen Juhl

Manager, Consumer Product Marketing
Maryjo Reynolds

Published by the American Academy of Pediatrics
141 Northwest Point Blvd, Elk Grove Village, IL 60007-1019
847/434-4000
Fax: 847/434-8000
www.aap.org

Cover design by Daniel Rembert
Book design by Linda Diamond

Library of Congress Control Number: 2011912900
ISBN: 978-1-58110-651-0

The recommendations in this publication do not indicate an exclusive course of treatment or serve as a standard of medical care. Variations, taking into account individual circumstances, may be appropriate.

The names and identifying details in each "A Parent's Story" may have been changed to protect the privacy of individuals. The content in these sections is for information only. The experiences may or may not be suitable for each family and do not indicate an exclusive course of treatment. Before starting any medical treatment or program, you should consult with your child's pediatrician, who can discuss your child's individual needs and counsel you about symptoms and treatment.

Products are mentioned for informational purposes only. Inclusion in this publication does not imply endorsement by the American Academy of Pediatrics. The American Academy of Pediatrics is not responsible for the content of the resources mentioned in this publication. Web site addresses are as current as possible, but may change at any time.

Every effort is made to keep *Autism Spectrum Disorders: What Every Parent Needs to Know* consistent with the most recent advice and information available from the American Academy of Pediatrics.

CB0070
9-321   1 2 3 4 5 6 7 8 9 10

What People Are Saying

Parents are craving knowledge and understanding of autism spectrum disorders and this guide is a wonderful resource to build that knowledge and encourage parents to advocate so that their child lives in a world where the dignity of every person is cherished, respected, and empowered.

Timothy P. Shriver, PhD

Chairman and CEO, Special Olympics

Covers a wide range of topics in a straightforward, commonsense manner, such as diagnosis, different behavioral therapies, family stress issues, and lots of other vital information. Essential reading for parents of young children with autism.

Temple Grandin

Author, *Thinking in Pictures: My Life With Autism*

Outstanding book and a tremendous resource for parents of children with autism spectrum disorders. It is also a must-read for anyone else working to help children with autism reach their full potential. The AAP and the book's editors, pediatricians Drs Alan Rosenblatt and Paul Carbone (who also happens to be the parent of a child with autism), know what they're talking about!

Richard E. Besser, MD, FAAP

Chief Health and Medical Editor, *ABC News*

Parents looking for a resource after an autism diagnosis will pull *Autism Spectrum Disorders: What Every Parent Needs to Know* off the shelf with great frequency. The AAP and Drs Carbone and Rosenblatt cover complex issues in an accessible manner. I will recommend this resource to families in need of quality information regarding services and supports for their children with autism.

Patricia Wright, PhD, MPH

National Director, Autism Services, Easter Seals

Autism Spectrum Disorders: What Every Parent Needs to Know is a must-read for every parent with a child on the autism spectrum. How you as a parent can help your child through play, language encouragement, structure, planning and partnering with professionals is outlined at each developmental stage from infancy through adulthood. Chapters on family relationships, your relationship with your pediatrician, and ways that you can become involved as an advocate for both your own child and for systems change, guide and encourage. Stories from multiple families, told in their own words, describe personal experiences and coping strategies that provide hope and comfort throughout the book. Get this book—it's a complete gem!

> Nora Wells, MEd
> Director of Programs, Family Voices

Instead of reading like a book, going through the pages of *Autism Spectrum Disorders: What Every Parent Needs to Know* is like having a casual conversation in your living room with a guru on ASD. The chapters on family, advocacy, and resources are particularly unique and helpful. The information is accurate, comprehensive, well organized, written in a compassionate, reader-friendly style, and interlaced with inspiring stories and endearing humor. Most parents will resonate with some of the stories; many will resonate with all of them. Some stories will bring tears and smiles at the same time. It is a must-have book for parents, service providers, and advocates alike.

> Chris Plauché Johnson, MEd, MA, MD, FAAP
> Medical Director, Autism Community Network; clinical
> professor (retired), University of Texas Health Science Center
> at San Antonio; cochair, American Academy of Pediatrics
> Autism Subcommittee (2003–2007)

Acknowledgments

Editors

Alan I. Rosenblatt, MD, FAAP

Paul S. Carbone, MD, FAAP

American Academy of Pediatrics
Board of Directors Reviewer

Sara H. Goza, MD, FAAP

American Academy of Pediatrics
Lead Staff

Carolyn Kolbaba

Manager, Consumer Publishing

Division of Product Development

Stephanie Mucha Skipper, MPH

Manager, Children With Special Needs
    Initiatives

Division of Children With Special Needs

Holly Kaminski

Coordinator, Product Development

Division of Product Development

Medical Reviewers/Contributors

Carolyn Bridgemohan, MD, FAAP

Charles Cowan, MD, FAAP

Larry Desch, MD, FAAP

Ellen Roy Elias, MD, FAAP

Kathryn Ellerbeck, MD, MPH, FAAP

Susan L. Hyman, MD, FAAP

Susan E. Levy, MD, FAAP

Patricia Manning-Courtney, MD, FAAP

Georgina Peacock, MD, MPH, FAAP

Marshalyn Yeargin-Allsopp, MD, FAAP

Parent Reviewers/Contributors

Beth Bullen, RN

Kate Clemont

Debra L. Dunn, Esq

Amy Kelly

Amy Kratchman

Bernadette Lionetta

Sharon A. Nagel, MSW, RSW

Chinyere Obimba

Melissa Parrish

Lee Stickle

Sandy Tiahrt, MS

Michelle Zier, JD

Additional Assistance

James G. Pawelski

Dan Walter

Writer

Winnie Yu

From the Editors

We dedicate this book to the children and families who inspire, teach, and challenge us daily to seek better answers and solutions.

Dr Rosenblatt thanks his wife, Lisa, and his children, Galit and Shachar, for the blessings and miracles that have led to this moment.

Dr Carbone thanks his wife, Katie, for her love, support, and understanding and also thanks Ben, for being the most wonderful son he could have ever hoped for.

❧ ❧ ❧ ❧ ❧

On behalf of the Council on Children With Disabilities Autism Subcommittee, we honor the many contributions of our colleague and friend, Gregory Stephen Liptak, MD, MPH, FAAP (1947–2012), to the field of children with special needs.

Table of Contents

Foreword

The American Academy of Pediatrics (AAP) welcomes you to the latest book in its parenting series, *Autism Spectrum Disorders: What Every Parent Needs to Know.*

Pediatricians are the first to see developmental concerns, so it is fitting that the AAP develop a book on autism spectrum disorders (ASDs) for parents and caregivers. In this book, parents will learn how ASDs are defined and diagnosed, and the types of behavioral and developmental therapies available for treating them. Stories from other parents will help them understand that they are not alone on this journey. This book will help parents understand how ASDs will affect their children as they grow older.

Pediatricians who specialize in ASDs have extensively reviewed this book. Under the direction of our editors, the material in this book was developed with the assistance of numerous reviewers and contributors. Because medical information is constantly changing, every effort has been made to ensure that this book contains the most up-to-date findings. Readers may want to visit the AAP Web site for parents, HealthyChildren.org, to keep current on this and other subjects.

It is the hope of the AAP that this book will become an invaluable resource and reference guide to parents. We are confident that parents and caregivers will find the book extremely valuable. We encourage its use along with the advice and counsel of our readers' pediatricians, who will provide individual guidance and assistance related to the health of children.

The AAP is an organization of 60,000 primary care pediatricians, pediatric medical subspecialists, and pediatric surgical specialists dedicated to the health, safety, and well-being of infants, children, adolescents, and young adults. *Autism Spectrum Disorders: What Every Parent Needs to Know* is part of ongoing AAP educational efforts to provide parents and caregivers with high-quality information on a broad spectrum of children's health issues.

Errol R. Alden, MD, FAAP
Executive Director/CEO
American Academy of Pediatrics

CHAPTER 1

What Are Autism Spectrum Disorders?

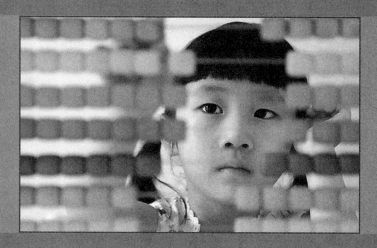

As a pediatrician whose son has an autism spectrum disorder (ASD), I (Dr Carbone) know all too well about the difficult emotions that often surround a diagnosis of an ASD. My son was diagnosed with an ASD in 2004 at the age of 2. Before the diagnosis, we were concerned about his development, beginning in infancy. At times he seemed uncomfortable with symptoms of acid reflux, and at other times he was extremely quiet and hard to engage. While he has always made forward progress, he reached his developmental milestones later than other children. For example, as a young toddler, he had difficulty using gestures, like pointing, to tell us what he wanted, and didn't begin to talk until he was 24 months old.

While getting the diagnosis was painful, it ultimately helped me to better understand him. It also began the process of knowing how to help him reach his potential.

Although his mother and I are pediatricians, we went through a grieving process just like any parents. At first I thought about the things I did with my father that my son and I might not be able to do, like playing sports. I later realized that although there are some things that are challenging for him, there are many things we do together that bring us both much joy. I have learned during this journey that parenting a child with an ASD is not "better" or "worse" than parenting any other child. It is simply different. My son has helped me appreciate and enjoy those differences.

We have always focused on what our son *can* do and not on what he can't. Along the way, we have tried to obtain the best therapies possible that allow him to reach even higher. As scientists, we knew that the best evidence-based therapy available for children with ASDs was behavioral therapy, so we began his behavioral therapy program while he was very young. In addition to intensive behavioral therapy, we were open to trying complementary and alternative therapies as long as they were safe. After doing some research, we tried a few different nutritional supplements and the gluten-free/casein-free (GFCF) diet, understanding that there was limited evidence that these treatments would help reduce the symptoms of autism. After some time we came to the conclusion that his progress with behavioral therapy was no better with these interventions than without them, and so we discontinued them. We have continued to support him with ongoing behavioral therapy and have been delighted with his progress.

Now our son is an active participant in his community. With the support of family, friends, educators, therapists, and doctors he enjoys many of the same activities of his peers: swimming, basketball, bowling, summer camp, reading, and discovering. All who take the time to get to know him are drawn in by his gentle demeanor, curious nature, and wonderful sense of humor.

❧ ❧ ❧ ❧ ❧

Ellen had always taken pride in her son's intelligence, his expansive vocabulary, and his knowledge of dinosaurs. But at 11, Brian was struggling socially. Classmates found his all-consuming obsession with dinosaurs annoying, and Brian grew impatient with them if they didn't know as much as he did about the prehistoric creatures. He had trouble understanding sarcasm from his peers. He couldn't tell when they were being mean but got overly sensitive when they weren't. He thought nothing of making rude, sarcastic comments during class while the teacher was talking.

Brian also behaved in unusual ways. He was always touching people when he was stuck waiting in lines, falling down at unexpected times, and making loud, inappropriate comments about people within earshot. What concerned Ellen the most was that Brian never seemed to look her in the eye while she was talking to him.

Over time, Ellen grew suspicious that something else was going on with her son, especially when she went back to college to get a degree in psychology and started doing more reading. Though he had already been diagnosed with attention-deficit/hyperactivity disorder (ADHD) at age 7, she began to wonder if he also had an ASD, a diagnosis that a teacher had once suggested but that Ellen had always dismissed. "He didn't fit the profile of what I thought was autism," she says. "I always thought children with autism were unattached, unresponsive, and in their own world."

Ellen had Brian evaluated by a psychologist. A screening test suggested that he had *high-functioning autism*, a form of ASD marked by an obsession with 1 or 2 topics, challenges with the social aspects of language, and difficulties navigating social relationships. The more she learned about high-functioning autism, the more Ellen was convinced that Brian had it. So far, Ellen has been hesitant about getting a formal diagnosis. She fears that the label will create a lifelong stigma for her son. "And I'm afraid some people will look at me and think I'm a bad parent," she says. (Ellen, Price, UT)

🐾 🐾 🐾 🐾 🐾

Chances are, you're familiar with some of the concerns that Ellen is facing or the difficult emotions that Dr Carbone has experienced while raising a child with an ASD. Like Ellen, you may be wondering whether you should have your child diagnosed or what a diagnosis will mean for your child's life. Like Dr Carbone, you may be looking for information about where to find help for your child's language delays, social challenges, and behavioral problems. Or maybe you suspect your child has an ASD but haven't addressed your concern with your pediatrician yet.

We hope that reading this book will help provide you with the information you are seeking to make the best decisions for your child. In this book, you will learn how ASDs are defined and diagnosed, and the types of behavioral and developmental therapies available for treating them. You will learn when medications may be required, and whether complementary and integrative medicine may be helpful. We will also help you create a treatment team that includes your pediatrician, and provide information to help you care for your child and get a handle on the types of services and assistance available to him. In addition, we will help you understand the effect of ASDs on you and the rest of your family. Stories from other parents will help you understand that you are not alone on this journey. You will acquire an understanding of how ASDs will affect your child as he grows older and the types of advocacy you can do as the most important part of the treatment team: the parent of a child with an ASD.

🐾 🐾 🐾 🐾 🐾

Autism spectrum disorders are a group of biologically based neurodevelopmental disorders that affect a child's behavior and social and communication skills. They belong to a group of disorders known as *pervasive developmental disorders* (PDDs), a distinction that includes ASDs, Asperger syndrome, and pervasive developmental disorder–not otherwise specified (PDD-NOS). These subcategories were used in the fourth edition of the *Diagnostic and Statistical Manual of Mental Disorders (DSM-IV),* a manual published by the American Psychiatric Association to provide diagnostic criteria for behavioral conditions. They will be eliminated in the new *DSM-5,* which will be published in 2013. You will read more about the differences later in this chapter.

For most children, these conditions are chronic and require lifelong management. Some children—approximately 3% to 25%, according to studies—improve over time to a point where they no longer meet diagnostic criteria for ASDs. In general, these children are the ones who have typical learning abilities and have received behavioral therapy (see Chapter 4). However, most children who improve still have other developmental and behavioral symptoms.

No doubt, we certainly hear a great deal about ASDs these days. A study by the Centers for Disease Control and Prevention (CDC) estimated that ASDs affect 1 in 88 children, about 1% of all children. Boys are 5 times as likely to be affected as girls, and white children are more often diagnosed than African American and Hispanic children.

A major reason for the dramatic increase in the diagnosis of ASDs has to do with changes in the way the conditions are diagnosed. In 1994, the diagnosis was changed to include children with milder symptoms, including those whose language is closer to normal cognitive milestones. In addition, a growing body of research showing the importance of early, intensive behavioral treatment in helping children with ASDs prompted the federal government to emphasize early detection, so that more children could receive services at a younger age. The emphasis on importance of early diagnosis and intervention inspired several major public education campaigns to teach parents about ASDs and the importance of early diagnosis.

In spite of all the public interest in and attention on autism, figuring out whether your child has an ASD is not easy. These conditions are remarkably complex and difficult to diagnose. No 2 children exhibit the same symptoms, and severity varies widely. Some cases may be subtle, while others may be more straightforward. In most cases, the process of determining

---

CAN A CHILD EVER FULLY RECOVER FROM AN AUTISM SPECTRUM DISORDER?

Symptoms of an autism spectrum disorder vary greatly from one child to the next. While it's possible for some children—studies range from 3% to 25%—to improve to the point where they no longer meet diagnostic criteria, most continue to have some degree of developmental or behavioral symptoms.

whether a child has an ASD usually begins with parents who are concerned about their child's development. But in some cases, the early sign of an ASD first comes to the attention of a pediatrician or child care provider who observes something different in the way the child plays, learns, speaks, or acts.

We'll discuss more about diagnosis in Chapter 3. First, we'll go back in time to see how autism emerged as a major health concern.

A Brief History of Autism

Autism was first described in 1943 by Dr Leo Kanner, a child psychiatrist at Johns Hopkins University School of Medicine. It was Dr Kanner who first coined the term *autism,* borrowed from the Swiss psychiatrist Eugen Bleuler, who used the word to describe the idiosyncratic, self-centered thinking he saw in schizophrenia. Kanner used *autism* to describe 11 children in his practice who seemed to prefer isolation to social engagement. The children all displayed extreme aloofness and total indifference to other people. They made little eye contact and did not engage in imaginary play. Some displayed an amazing ability for rote memory. Others were obsessed with routines, spinning toys, and mechanical objects. Dr Kanner believed that autism was an inborn disorder and that children with this condition entered the world without biological underpinnings for social interaction. These were children who lived in their own world. Even today, Dr Kanner's descriptions of autism are highly regarded and considered some of the best ever written.

FASCINATING FACT

Donald Triplett, the first child cited in Dr Kanner's now-famous report on autism, was profiled in *The Atlantic* in October 2010. At the time, he was 77, living in Forest, MS. Although he faced many challenges throughout his life, he was embraced by his community and enjoyed doing activities such as playing golf. Read his story online at www.theatlantic.com/magazine/archive/2010/10/autism-8217-s-first-child/8227.

In the 1950s, Freudian psychoanalysts put a new spin on autism, contending that the condition resulted from the emotional withdrawal of a baby born to a cold and emotionally distant parent. In particular, they focused on mothers and called these parents "refrigerator mothers." Bruno Bettelheim, then the director of the Orthogenic School in Chicago, became fascinated with children who had autism and advanced this theory. (Bettelheim had a PhD in philosophy but was widely cited as a child psychologist. He lectured on psychology at the University of Chicago, despite the lack of any formal training.) Bettelheim's most famous patient was a boy named Joey, whom he described in 1959 as a "mechanical boy" in the popular magazine *Scientific American.* At 18 months, Joey was unable to speak and was described by his grandparents as "remote and inaccessible." Joey became fascinated with mechanical objects and learned to take apart and reassemble an electric fan. By the age of 4, Joey was spending a great deal of his time rocking back and forth and becoming completely consumed with mechanical objects.

Like many of his colleagues at the time, Bettelheim blamed Joey's unusual behaviors on his parents. Bettelheim claimed that their aloof parenting style forced Joey to withdraw into his own world and marked the beginning of his descent into schizophrenia. In fact, autism was classified as a form of childhood schizophrenia in the first 2 editions of *DSM.*

Bettelheim's views persisted for years until experts began to consider autism from more biological perspectives. In 1964, a research psychologist named Bernard Rimland described infantile autism as a neurologic disorder with a strong genetic component. Rimland and his wife were personally acquainted with autism—they were the parents of a child with autism, whom they had diagnosed themselves.

Studies in the early 1970s showed that despite similar symptoms, autism was a disorder distinct from childhood schizophrenia. In 1977, the first study of twins and autism was published in the *Journal of Child Psychology and Psychiatry.* The study found a strong genetic influence in identical twins who had autism. If one twin had autism, the other twin was much more likely to have other cognitive differences too. Finding a genetic connection to autism meant that autism needed to be described more precisely so that it could be properly studied and better understood. That became possible in 1980, when *infantile autism* finally received its own separate category in the third edition of *DSM.*

EARLY SIGNS OF AUTISM SPECTRUM DISORDERS

Social Differences

- Resists snuggling when picked up; arches back instead
- May have temperament differences during infancy, such as being described as a very quiet or very fussy baby
- Makes little or no eye contact
- Shows no or less expression in response to parent's smile or other facial expressions
- May avoid following a parent's gaze or finger to see what parent is looking at or pointing to
- No or less pointing to objects or events to get parents to look at them
- Less likely to bring objects to show to parents just to share his interest
- Less likely to show appropriate facial expressions
- Difficulty in recognizing what others might be thinking or feeling by looking at their facial expressions
- Less likely to show concern (empathy) for others
- Has difficulty in establishing and keeping friendships

Communication Differences

- Says no single words by 15 months or 2-word phrases by 24 months
- May repeat exactly what others say without understanding its meaning (parroting or echolalia)
- Responds to sounds (like a car horn or a cat's meow) but less likely to respond to name being called
- May refer to self as "you" and others as "I" (pronoun reversal)
- Shows no or less interest in communicating
- Less likely to start or continue a conversation
- Less likely to use toys or other objects to represent people or real life in pretend play
- May have a good rote memory, especially for numbers, songs, TV jingles, or a specific topic
- May lose language milestones, usually between the ages of 15 and 24 months in some children (regression)

Behavioral Differences (Stereotypic, Repetitive, and Restricted Patterns)

- May rock, spin, sway, twirl fingers, or flap hands (stereotypic behavior)
- Likes routines, order, and rituals
- May be obsessed with a few activities, doing them repeatedly during the day
- More likely to play with parts of toys instead of the whole toy (for example, spinning wheels of a toy truck)

(continued on next page)

EARLY SIGNS OF AUTISM SPECTRUM DISORDERS, CONTINUED

Behavioral Differences (Stereotypic, Repetitive, and Restricted Patterns), *continued*

- May have splinter skills, such as the ability to read at an early age but often without understanding what it means
- May not cry if in pain or seem to have any fear
- May be very sensitive or not sensitive at all to smells, sounds, lights, textures, and touch (sensory processing differences)
- May have unusual use of vision or gaze (for example, looks at objects from unusual angles)
- May have unusual or intense but narrow interests

WHAT AN AUTISM SPECTRUM DISORDER MIGHT LOOK LIKE

It isn't always easy for parents to know if a child has an autism spectrum disorder (ASD). Some of the symptoms of ASDs may be seen in children with other types of developmental or behavioral problems or, to a lesser extent, in children with typical development. Also, not all of the symptoms are seen in all children. Some children may only display a few of the symptoms. This is what makes the process of diagnosing ASDs difficult. But here are some examples that may help distinguish a child with an ASD from other children.

At 12 Months

A child with typical development will turn his head when he hears his name.

A child with an ASD might not turn to look, even after his name is repeated several times, but will respond to other sounds.

At 18 Months

A child with delayed speech skills will point, gesture, or use facial expressions to make up for her lack of talking.

A child with an ASD might make no attempt to compensate for delayed speech or might limit speech to parroting what is heard on TV or what she just heard.

At 24 Months

A child without an ASD brings a picture to show his mother and shares his joy from it with her.

A child with an ASD might bring her a bottle of bubbles to open but doesn't look at his mom's face when he does or share in the pleasure of playing together.

Defining Autism Spectrum Disorders Today

Even now, as we go to press, the definition of ASDs is evolving. To understand how it will change, we need to look at *DSM-IV*, which was published in 1994, and the soon-to-be published *DSM-5*, which is in the process of being written. In short, the disorder remains unchanged, but how it is classified and described will be different.

In *DSM-IV*, ASDs are listed as 1 of 5 PDDs. The other PDDs are Asperger syndrome, PDD-NOS, childhood disintegrative disorder, and Rett syndrome. Here is how these conditions are defined.

Autistic Spectrum Disorder

Autistic spectrum disorder is what most people know as autism. Children who have ASDs have problems relating to others socially. They may have trouble making eye contact, building friendships, and sharing things they enjoy with other people. As infants, they often display limited or no *joint attention,* a behavior that involves enjoying an object or event with another person by looking back and forth between the two.

Many children with ASDs have delayed language skills or use language in ways that are out of the ordinary. Rather than use language to connect with others, they may use words to meet basic needs, or they may just use their vocabulary for labeling but not to indicate their needs. For instance, a child may have a vocabulary of 20 or more words for labeling objects yet not be able to use those words to ask for an item at an appropriate time. In some cases, children may not develop the ability to use verbal communication.

While social difficulties may appear in the first year, communication problems may not become obvious until the second year. A 2-year-old may lack words to communicate or may not be able to use the words he does have for meaningful interaction, and by age 3, may have no phrases or sentences. Over time, these communication challenges become even more noticeable. Some children may have trouble knowing how to start a conversation. Others may have echolalia, in which they repeat what people say to them. Still others may constantly recite scripts from favorite videos or TV shows.

When children with ASDs play, they rarely use their imagination. They may not act out scenarios or pretend that an object is something else (using a pencil for a laser sword or a banana for a telephone, for instance). When they do play, they may prefer to arrange their toys or play with parts of a toy—opening doors on a car door instead of driving it, for example. Some children form attachments to hard objects such as a ballpoint pen or flashlight instead of stuffed animals.

Children with ASDs may become rigidly fixated on topics that most other people would consider unusual and have trouble letting go of these topics. For instance, they may be interested in movie credits, license plates, or addresses.

Some may become consumed with following rigid routines that may not have any useful purpose or have a strong insistence on sameness. For example, children with ASDs may prefer that certain activities be done in a precise order and may become highly anxious if a routine or ritual is broken. Likewise, they may have difficulty with transitions if they have not been prepared ahead of time.

In addition, children with ASDs may engage in motor activities that appear unusual and to serve no purpose. These may include hand flapping, rocking in place, or walking on tiptoe. Some children become unusually intrigued with parts of objects rather than the objects themselves.

Most of these problems will emerge before the age of 3. According to the current *DSM,* diagnosing an ASD involves first ruling out 2 other PDDs that we will discuss on page 14, Rett syndrome and childhood disintegrative disorder.

Asperger Syndrome

Asperger syndrome is named for Hans Asperger, an Austrian pediatrician. In 1944, Asperger—who did not know about Dr Kanner's work—published an article describing children whose symptoms were much like those Dr Kanner detailed. But the children Asperger described were typical in their verbal and cognitive skills.

Children with Asperger syndrome share traits with those who have ASDs. Both groups have difficulties with social interactions. They often have trouble looking people in the eye, rarely use gestures or facial expressions, and have trouble knowing how close to stand to others. They also may have less interest in engaging others and may not share objects or experiences of interest with others.

Like children with ASDs, those with Asperger syndrome may fixate on narrow interests, sometimes to the exclusion of other topics. They may prefer rituals and routines, and may become anxious and upset when those are altered or disrupted. They may also engage in repetitive behaviors such as spinning or rocking for long periods. Children with Asperger syndrome may become preoccupied with parts of objects too.

A key difference, however, is in language skills. Early language milestones are not delayed in children with Asperger syndrome. In fact, these children may even be early readers who speak in an overly formal way and have an impressive vocabulary. Some may affectionately be referred to as "little professors." Even so, their language skills may be quite unique or different. They may talk continuously about a limited number of topics; have difficulty understanding certain types of humor, figures of speech, and jokes; and have less understanding of the social use of language, such as how to start and maintain a conversation or how to end one.

Another difference is that children with Asperger syndrome do not have cognitive delays, which may or may not occur in autism. The *DSM* specifies that children with Asperger syndrome are also capable of doing age-appropriate self-help skills like bathing and dressing and will be curious about their environment in childhood.

Pervasive Developmental Disorder–Not Otherwise Specified

A child may be diagnosed with PDD-NOS when she has some of the signs and symptoms of ASDs or Asperger syndrome but doesn't meet the strict criteria used to diagnose those conditions. Children with PDD-NOS may have poor social skills because of limited verbal or nonverbal skills, or persistent and repetitive interests, activities, and behaviors. But they differ from children with ASDs or Asperger syndrome in that their symptoms may not appear until they are older.

Some people feel that PDD-NOS is a subthreshold or atypical form of ASD because children who have it show certain symptoms but not others. For instance, a child may have difficulties with social interactions and communication but have no persistent, repetitive behaviors. Symptoms may also be milder. Still, *DSM* specifies that PDD-NOS involves a "severe and pervasive impairment" in developing social skills. This means it can create many of the same challenges as ASDs and Asperger syndrome. This may be especially true if the child also has an intellectual disability that affects her cognitive functioning or other behavioral challenges, such as ADHD.

Childhood Disintegrative Disorder

Childhood disintegrative disorder is a rare disorder that affects 2 in 100,000 children. The condition is also known as Heller syndrome. Children with childhood disintegrative disorder develop normally until age 2 or 3, then lose social skills, expressive or receptive language, play skills, motor skills, or bowel and bladder control. They will go on to have difficulties with social interactions or communication and may also develop stereotyped behaviors seen with ASDs. Because childhood disintegrative disorder is so similar to ASD with regression (see box on next page), it has been proposed that it be eliminated from *DSM-5*.

Rett Syndrome

Also known as Rett disorder, Rett syndrome is a genetic condition that causes behavioral changes that may initially look like ASDs. An infant with Rett syndrome has typical development and head circumference until about 5 months of age, when growth in head size may begin to slow and early motor skills start to disappear. Most children develop repetitive hand movements like tapping, wringing, and clapping. They also have trouble with gross motor skills and may lose the ability to walk. Rett syndrome is a possible cause of ASDs. It occurs primarily in girls and usually appears before age 2 years. Rett syndrome will likely not be included in *DSM-5* as a subtype of ASDs. See Chapter 2 for a more detailed description of this syndrome.

My son is 20 months old and was developing normally until recently. Someone suggested he might be regressing to an autism spectrum disorder (ASD). What does that mean?

Regression occurs in about 25% of children with ASDs. These children may appear to develop normally, then experience a gradual or sudden loss of social or communication skills. Studies suggest that this is most likely to occur between 18 and 24 months. They may stop talking if they've already started using words and stop turning their heads when their names are called. They may withdraw into their own world and appear more distant and less interested in their surroundings. They may become more irritable. For parents, the abrupt change is alarming.

A close look at children's behavior before diagnosis shows that some of the delays in developmental milestones might have been present before regression, at least to a mild degree. When researchers looked at the home videos of these children at their first birthday parties, they saw subtle signs in some children before regression became obvious and an ASD was detected. The most common sign they noticed was that these children did not consistently turn their heads when their names were called.

The New Definition

In the new *DSM-5*, due out in 2013, it's been proposed that a single diagnostic category for ASDs replace the PDDs category. All children who have ASDs, Asperger syndrome, childhood disintegrative disorder, or PDD-NOS will be consolidated under the single diagnosis of ASD, and those other terms will be eliminated. The new *DSM-5* will provide a simplified way of defining autism.

To be diagnosed with an ASD in *DSM-5*, a child must have problems in 2 main areas, social forms of communication and repetitive behaviors. More specifically, these are

- Persistent struggles with social communication and social interactions in various situations that cannot be explained by developmental delays. These may include problems with give-and-take in normal conversations, difficulties making eye contact, a lack of facial expressions, and difficulties adjusting behaviors to fit different social situations.
- Obsessive and repetitive patterns of behavior, interests, or activities. These may include unusual and constant movements, strong attachment to rituals and routines, and fixations on unusual objects and interests. These may also include sensory abnormalities,

which have always been commonly seen in children with ASDs but are not used currently to diagnose an ASD or Asperger syndrome. Children with sensory abnormalities may be hypersensitive to certain sounds, textures, or lights. They may also be unusually insensitive to things in the environment that usually cause pain, heat, or cold.

The new criteria note that symptoms must begin in early childhood and disrupt a child's day-to-day functioning. In addition, diagnosis must take into account an individual's age, stage of development, intellectual abilities, and language level.

If you have any concerns about the diagnosis your child receives or questions about *DSM* classification or terminology, talk with your child's pediatrician.

What We Know and Don't Know

We're a long way from the days when Bruno Bettelheim blamed parents for a child's autism. We now know that it is a neurodevelopmental disorder, something that occurs in the early formation of the brain. We also know the importance of early diagnosis and treatment, and now have the tools to help us determine whether a child has or is at risk for ASDs. To that end, organizations like the CDC and American Academy of Pediatrics have waged successful public awareness campaigns like "Learn the Signs. Act Early." (www.cdc.gov/actearly) that have promoted surveillance and screening leading to early diagnosis. This has made early treatment possible for the benefit of millions of children. In addition, we know that certain therapies are more effective than others at treating symptoms.

For example, developmental and behavioral interventions are the mainstay of supporting individuals with ASDs. Behavioral interventions focus on changing specific behaviors and symptoms. As these behaviors change, social relationships and mastery of basic developmental capacities improve. There are several different types of behavioral interventions (see Chapter 4). Studies have consistently shown that children with ASDs who use intensive and systematic behavioral principles to reinforce developmentally appropriate skills have improved social communication, intelligence, language, behavior, and self-help skills when compared with children with ASDs who did not.

Throughout this book we discuss resources and services available today that did not exist just a few years ago and provide strategies on how to access them. People with special needs are more widely accepted in today's society, and the desire to include them in family and community life has opened doors and allowed them to participate in activities and go to venues that were previously inaccessible. Children born with ASDs today have greater hope for full and rewarding lives than they ever did in previous generations.

Even so, there are still many unknowns. The exact cause of the condition, for instance, has not been determined, although it is now clear that ASD has many different causes, some of which can be identified. In addition, all children with ASDs are unique, so there is no single treatment that works for every child. While scientists do know that the rate of ASD diagnosis is rising rapidly, they have yet to figure out the rate at which ASD itself is increasing. The search for answers has led to unfounded theories and unproven remedies.

Take vaccines. Research shows that almost 20% of parents worry that vaccines are not safe for their children and might lead to health problems like autism or diabetes. In particular, some people worry about the measles-mumps-rubella (MMR) vaccine. Their belief is bolstered by the fact that regression in children later diagnosed with ASDs might occur weeks to months after the MMR vaccine is given. The timing has led many parents to mistakenly assume a cause-and-effect relationship between the MMR vaccine and ASDs. Research has long since shown that vaccines do not cause ASDs, but unfortunately, the concern about an association still persists. (For more detailed information, see Chapter 2.)

Many people also worried about thimerosal, a mercury-based preservative used in vaccines to prevent bacterial contamination. That fear was also proven false. Since 2001, most routine children's vaccines made in the United States have had no thimerosal except for some flu vaccines. But the rates at which ASDs have been diagnosed have continued to climb.

The search for a cause has also led to theories about abnormalities in the gastrointestinal (GI) tract causing changes in the brain. The belief that ASDs are a GI disorder has given rise to nutritional therapies that have limited scientific backing.

Of particular interest has been the GFCF diet. This diet is based on the belief that gluten (a molecule found in barley, rye, oats, and wheat) and casein (a molecule found in milk

---

My friend says her sister cured her son of autism with the gluten-free/casein-free (GFCF) diet. Should we try it?

Although the American Academy of Pediatrics does not endorse the GFCF diet, it does understand that some parents may want to consider trying it. Before doing so, it's important to discuss your child's nutritional needs with your pediatrician. For instance, a diet without casein restricts the amount of calcium and vitamin D a child gets and puts her at risk for osteoporosis later in life. Therefore, it's essential to find other ways to meet your child's needs for calcium, vitamin D, and iron. You also have to make sure your child meets her caloric needs. Your pediatrician might refer you to a registered dietitian.

Before going on the GFCF diet, make sure to identify target behaviors and how you will measure changes in those behaviors. By doing so, you will be able to gauge whether the diet is working. Finally, make sure to keep your child's food preferences and routines in mind. Children with ASDs are often resistant to change. And your child may not like the idea of eating foods that are different from what she's used to eating and what the rest of the family eats. You may need to use behavioral strategies to get her to eat new foods. If your child has improvement in irritability or intestinal symptoms but no change in symptoms of ASDs, it may be that she has a common intestinal problem like lactose intolerance.

---

products) cause substances produced by these foods to enter the bloodstream and travel to the brain, triggering symptoms we see as ASDs. You'll find more information on nutritional therapies and other alternative remedies in Chapter 7.

The Bottom Line

As the parent of a child who has an ASD—or a child whom you suspect has an ASD—you probably want to learn more about ASDs. In this book, we will do our best to provide you with the most up-to-date facts and information about ASDs. We'll also share stories from other parents, who are often the best sources of information as well as emotional support. Our goal is to empower you with the knowledge you need as you embark on this journey with your child. We encourage you to partner with your child's pediatrician, who can help you every step of the way. Armed with the appropriate facts and information, you will be able to make the best possible choices for your child. And that's reassuring for any parent.

Autism Champion: Carmen Pingree

Back in 1979, when Carmen Pingree's son Brian was diagnosed with autism, 95% of children with autism were institutionalized. The only program for children with autism near their home in Salt Lake City, UT, had 4 students in it, with 12 on a waiting list. And getting a diagnosis typically took years.

Even getting answers for Brian had been a struggle despite all the classic signs—Brian rocked for hours at a time, ignored the affection and attention of his family, and became fascinated with windshield wipers, heights, and lights. He had a penchant for unscrewing objects and undoing latches and locks. Experts labeled him "abused," "emotionally disturbed," and "mentally retarded."

When he was nearly 4 years old, he was finally diagnosed, much to Carmen's relief. "We finally had a name for what we were dealing with," she says. "We read books, attended conferences, met other parents, and found a small behavior therapy program with young dedicated professionals. The information lowered our frustration and gave us tools to work with Brian at home until we could find a way to expand the preschool program."

Together with other parents, Carmen obtained a school building that was being closed. Then she turned her energies toward getting funding from the Utah state legislature. She went back to college to get a master's degree in special education and political science, a perfect melding of the task that lay ahead. She invited legislators to visit the program, learn about autism, and hear budget requests over lunch.

Her husband and even her other 4 children got involved in the effort, which ultimately succeeded in securing funds for autism services in Utah, including the preschool program, an adolescent teaching home, and a residential treatment program.

Carmen didn't just lobby. She also began to pursue federal and community funding for autism research and helped create a 5-year joint epidemiologic and genetic study between the University of Utah and the University of California, Los Angeles. Through the years, she became an autism research consultant for Stanford University and Utah State University, the president of the Autism Society of Utah, and a frequent lecturer and researcher whose studies have appeared in numerous scientific journals.

When a new building was constructed in 2003 for the expanded preschool program (which by then included elementary-aged children with autism), it was named The Carmen B. Pingree Center for Children with Autism. An active research site, the center also offers support for parents and siblings of children with ASDs and serves as a training ground for graduate students specializing in ASDs, as well as pediatric and psychiatry residents.

Brian is in his thirties now, but Carmen continues to advocate for families with children with ASDs and serves on the advisory board of the center as well as the board of the program where her son resides. "Brian enjoys his role as uncle to the 20 Pingree grandchildren," Carmen says. "The whole family continues to involve Brian in their lives and to support programming for individuals with autism. They consider these opportunities for service a great blessing in their lives."

CHAPTER 2

What Causes Autism Spectrum Disorders?

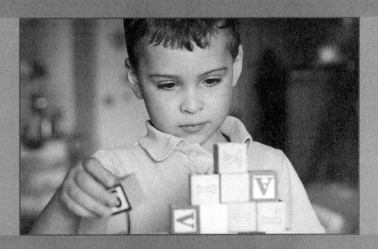

Chances are, you already knew someone with an autism spectrum disorder (ASD) before you learned or suspected that your child had one. Or maybe you knew someone who worked with children and adults who have ASDs. The number of children being diagnosed with an ASD has been rising steadily in recent decades. In fact, in early 2012, the Centers for Disease Control and Prevention (CDC) reported that the total number of ASD cases in a given population at a specific time had increased 78% in the short span of just 6 years. The CDC found that 1 in 88 children had an ASD in 2008, well above the rate of 1 in 110 that had been found in 2006. That meant that more than 1% of all children in the United States had an ASD.

The report gave credence to a study released in 2009 using the National Survey of Children's Health, which was conducted by interviewing parents in 2007. That study found that 1 in 91 children had been diagnosed with an ASD. Clearly, ASDs have become a major issue, one that prompted the authors of the CDC report to declare autism "an urgent public health concern."

The latest increase was not really news, though the extent of it certainly was. The reason for the increase, however, was—and remains—open to debate. Some of it, of course, can be traced to greater public awareness of the disorder and improvements in screening tools that have made parents and health care professionals alike more adept at spotting and identifying children with ASDs. Efforts like the "Learn the Signs. Act Early." campaign by the CDC and several efforts by the American Academy of Pediatrics have certainly made a difference. Intense media coverage and the publication of a growing body of research in professional journals have fueled that awareness too. Changes in diagnostic criteria that broadened the definition of an ASD also contributed to the surge. Since 1980, when autism first landed in the third edition of the *Diagnostic and Statistics Manual of Mental Disorders* as its own separate entity, criteria have been expanded to include milder cases of the condition such as Asperger syndrome and pervasive development disorder–not otherwise specified.

Legislative maneuvers had an effect too, namely passage of the Individuals with Disabilities Education Act (IDEA) in 1990. Before IDEA was enacted, children might have received educational classifications such as *intellectual disability, learning disability, speech or language impairment,* or *emotional disturbance* before they could be eligible for special education services. Once autism was recognized as an educational classification by IDEA, the numbers of children labeled with these other categories went down, while the number of children under the autism classification went up.

That same year, Congress passed the Americans with Disabilities Act, which required states to administer their programs for children with disabilities in the most integrated settings possible. This federal legislation led to closure of some institutions that once housed children with disabilities and instead encouraged local governments to support families who were raising their children at home. As a result, children with autism, especially those who also had other behavior problems and intellectual disability, began to attend public schools. Instead of being hidden away in institutions, these children were now being counted among those in special education programs.

But some experts have concluded that these factors account for only some of the increase. Changes in how an ASD is diagnosed, for instance, could explain only 25% of the rise in autism cases in California between 1992 and 2005, according to a study from Columbia University. That meant that 1 in 4 children diagnosed with an ASD today would not have been given that diagnosis in 1993. On the other hand, a recent study from England estimated the rate of ASDs in adults to be similar to that of children. This would seem to indicate that the true risk for developing an ASD is not increased for today's children. So while some recent events explain why an ASD diagnosis is made more often, there still is vigorous debate whether the true risk of a child having an ASD is increasing.

As part of this discussion, it's important to appreciate the difference between *an increased risk* for an ASD (such as older age of parents) and what *causes* the condition (ie, certain medical and genetic syndromes). A *risk factor,* such as parental age, does not directly cause an ASD but makes it more likely for the child to have an ASD compared with those without the risk factor. The increased risk for an ASD means that parental age is probably one factor among many that may contribute to the child's diagnosis but by itself is not the cause. In congenital rubella syndrome (see page 33), an infection during pregnancy with the rubella virus causes the ASD, whereas in fragile X syndrome (FXS) (see page 28), the cause of the ASD is a particular sequence of DNA on the X chromosome.

Challenges of Autism Spectrum Disorders

Truth is, we are just beginning to learn about what causes an ASD. In about 15% of children with an ASD, the condition is associated with a clear underlying cause such as a chromosome abnormality, a genetic syndrome, or a known environmental cause. In most children, however, the underlying cause of the ASD is not obvious.

What we do know about ASDs is that they are a group of biologically based neurodevelopmental disorders with a strong genetic component. In short, an ASD is the result of something that occurs in the development of the brain. Exactly what triggers the event (or events) in the brain is still not fully understood. Scientists are fairly certain that autism is the result of complex interaction between genetic risk and environmental exposure, but they do not yet know exactly how much is genetic and how much is environmental. It's also quite possible that there are several genetic factors being influenced by the environment. But these environmental risk factors are still poorly understood and have not been sufficiently identified yet. One thing scientists are certain about: ASDs come in many forms and have multiple causes. Understanding the causes of ASDs has been a major research challenge that as of now still eludes us.

Genetics of Autism Spectrum Disorders

To understand hereditary influences on autism, it helps to have some basic knowledge of genetics. Genetics is the study of heredity, the passing on of cellular instructions from parents to their offspring, which determine traits of the offspring such as hair color, eye color, and height. All our body cells have 46 chromosomes—2 sex chromosomes and 22 pairs of non-sex or autosomal chromosomes. We inherit half of our chromosomes from each of our parents. Chromosomes are made up of DNA, which is shaped like a double helix or spiral ladder. Genes are the units of DNA that code instructions for making proteins that enable each cell to do what it's assigned to do. In other words, genes provide body cells with instruction manuals on what they need to do to make our bodies function. Changes in DNA can affect how genes work. A change in an individual gene, called a mutation, can lead to certain diseases and disorders.

BRAIN ABNORMALITIES IN AUTISM SPECTRUM DISORDERS

Children with autism spectrum disorders (ASDs) have distinct differences in their brain that are not seen in children without ASDs. And while these differences don't explain the cause of ASDs, they do explain some of the social differences, language issues, and motor skill difficulties that children with ASDs often display.

Among the key differences are

- Larger than normal head size, also known as macrocephaly.
- Greater brain volume.
- Fewer number of Purkinje cells in the cerebellum. Purkinje cells are large neurons in the brain responsible for coordinating motor skills. Recent studies have shown they are also involved in language, attention, and mental imagery.
- Abnormal maturation of the forebrain limbic system. The limbic system is made up of several brain structures, including the hippocampus, amygdala, thalamic nuclei, and limbic cortex. These structures are associated with emotion, behavior, long-term memory, and smell.
- Abnormalities in the frontal and temporal lobes. The frontal lobes are involved in various aspects of higher cognitive functioning, control of emotions and behavioral impulses, as well as the ability to transform thoughts into words. The temporal lobes play an important role in auditory perception and processing, visual processing, and the formation of long-term memory. Sensations of touch and taste also seem to be integrated with memory in the temporal lobes.
- Brainstem abnormalities. The brainstem connects the brain to the spinal cord. It carries sensory signals from the body to the brain and motor signals from the brain back to the rest of the body. The brainstem is also involved in regulating cardiac and respiratory functions, the sleep cycle, and consciousness.
- Neocortical malformations. The neocortex is the thin outer layer of the brain involved in higher functions such as sensory perception, generation of motor commands, spatial reasoning, conscious thought, and language. Disruptions to normal formation of this region of the brain are also associated with intellectual disability and seizures.

Scientists know that many of these brain structures are formed during the first 2 trimesters of pregnancy. As a result, experts suspect that environmental influences that may contribute to the development of ASDs are most likely those that occur to the mother early in her pregnancy. Furthermore, newer brain imaging techniques suggest that there are atypical connections between different parts of the brain of individuals with ASDs. Future research will help us to understand the nature of these abnormal connections and how they affect the function of the brain in a manner that leads to symptoms of an ASD.

Scientists have known for decades that genetics play an important role in the development of ASDs. Identical twins, who share the same genes, are significantly more likely to both have an ASD than fraternal twins, who share fewer genes. According to a large study published in 2011, a younger sibling of a child with an ASD has approximately 20 times the risk of developing an ASD as a child who does not have an affected sibling. And gender plays an important role too, as boys are more likely to have an ASD than girls. In the 2011 study, approximately 1 in 4 younger male siblings developed an ASD, whereas 1 in 11 younger female siblings were diagnosed with an ASD by the age of 3 years.

Experts know too that there are many genetic abnormalities involved in ASDs, not just a single abnormality (as there is in, say, sickle cell anemia); none of these are in all children with an ASD. Some children with an ASD have genetic mutations—permanent changes in DNA—that they did not inherit from their parents. Some children have changes in the structure of their chromosomes. Other children with ASDs have deletions and duplications of genetic material. These genetic abnormalities—rare genetic mutations, chromosomal abnormalities, and deletions and duplications of genetic material—account for at least 10% of all cases of ASD. Down syndrome, for example, is caused by having an extra copy of chromosome 21, and children with this condition have a very high prevalence—almost 10%—of autism. But each genetic abnormality by itself is rare and occurs in no more than 1% to 2% of all ASD cases.

Because each of the many genetic factors that may increase the risk for an ASD account for such a small percentage of all cases, scientists suspect that there are other factors that have yet to be discovered at play. It's quite possible that ASDs, as with other conditions, are the result of a variety of interactions between genes and factors in the environment. Ongoing research will continue to identify genetic and environmental factors involved in the underlying causes of ASDs.

Genetic Disorders and Autism Spectrum Disorders

Some people diagnosed with an ASD have known genetic mutations that result in a specific genetic disorder. Not every child with one of these disorders has an ASD, but having one of these genetic disorders certainly raises a child's risk for developing ASD. A partial list of the many genetic disorders associated with ASDs follows.

Fragile X Syndrome

Fragile X syndrome is a genetic disorder that affects the X chromosome passed down on the mother's side. It is the most common known genetic cause of ASDs and intellectual disability in boys. Because boys have only one X chromosome, they are affected more severely than girls. Boys with FXS may have distinctive physical features that may include having an unusually large head, ears, and testicles (after puberty). Children with FXS may also have weak muscles and loose joints. Fragile X syndrome is the most common cause of *inherited* cognitive impairment, which can range from learning disabilities to more severe intellectual disabilities. As many as 30% to 50% of people with FXS will have some characteristics of ASDs.

If your child has an ASD and intellectual disability or global developmental delays—meaning your child isn't reaching all the developmental milestones that are expected at different ages—or there is a history of intellectual disability on the mother's side of the family, testing for FXS should be done.

Rett Syndrome

Rett syndrome occurs primarily in girls and usually appears sometime in the first 2 years of life after a period of normal development. Girls with Rett syndrome typically lose control of hand skills and develop hand-wringing movements. They also develop difficulties walking, slowed head growth, seizures, and trouble with social skills.

Thanks to DNA sequencing, Rett syndrome can be diagnosed in more than 90% of cases.

Tuberous Sclerosis Complex

Children who have tuberous sclerosis complex have lesions in the brain, skin, and other organs. The condition is often associated with recurrent seizures. The link to ASDs in tuberous sclerosis complex is high—as many as 25% of children with this condition have an ASD.

Angelman Syndrome

Angelman syndrome affects 1 in 15,000 children. Children who have this disorder have intellectual disability, an unsteady gait, atypical laughter, seizures, and distinctive facial features. The condition is often overlooked as a cause of ASDs, intellectual disability, or cerebral palsy. Certain genetic tests can identify more than 80% of cases.

Phenylketonuria

Universal newborn screening has almost eliminated this once common cause of intellectual disability and ASDs. Phenylketonuria is a metabolic disorder that affects the body's ability to process a specific chemical called phenylalanine, which is found in many foods. When the chemical builds up in the body, it can become toxic to the developing brain. Restricting foods that contain phenylalanine in early infancy can prevent disabilities.

Smith-Lemli-Opitz Syndrome

Smith-Lemli-Opitz syndrome (SLOS) is a rare disorder caused by a defect in the way cholesterol is manufactured. It affects 1 in 20,000 children. Children with this condition often have multiple congenital malformations, such as cleft palate, extra toes, and genital deformities. However, some children with mild SLOS have an ASD and mild webbing of their toes. They may experience failure to thrive and feeding problems. Most children with this condition are on the autism spectrum.

GENETIC TESTS

New genetic tests called *microarray* allow geneticists to see extremely tiny changes in DNA. Over time these tests are becoming more sensitive and one day may give us a better understanding of how changes in DNA cause autism spectrum disorders.

Could Epigenetics Have the Answer?

Epigenetics merges nature and nurture. It is the study of how the environment changes the way genes work. Epigenetic changes occur on the surface of genes and may be caused by exposure to environmental factors in the foods you eat and stress you experience. Scientists believe it's possible that these epigenetic changes are passed on from one generation to the next.

Most often, these epigenetic changes result from methyl groups, chemical entities that latch on to DNA and then silence or activate the gene. Some experts believe that epigenetics may eventually help researchers pinpoint the potential environmental causes of autism, as well as many other diseases (for example, cancer, Alzheimer, obesity), and lead to the development of new therapies for treatment. Epigenetic factors are already known to cause certain genetic disorders such as Angelman syndrome (see page 29).

Among recent findings using epigenetics is a study of oxytocin. Experts have long suspected that people with ASDs do not have as much oxytocin (the bonding hormone responsible for social behavior such as recognizing loved ones, building trust in others, and alleviating anxiety) as those without ASDs. Recent research from scientists at Duke University has shown that the problem may actually lie with oxytocin receptors, which allow the hormone to bind to neurons and take effect. The researchers found that people with an ASD have more methyl groups on the oxytocin receptor gene than people without an ASD. When these methyl groups become part of the genetic code, it is believed that the gene is "turned off," which would explain some of the social difficulties in people with ASDs. Controlling methylation of these genes may possibly lead to new treatments, but more research is still needed before that can occur.

Environmental Causes

No one knows exactly what it is in our environment that may lead to an ASD, but there have been no shortage of theories as to a probable cause. Some people, for instance, point to vaccines, especially if their child displayed no signs of ASDs until after he received the vaccine, despite evidence to the contrary that has shown no link.

Three main theories that have been raised about vaccines and autism are

1. The measles-mumps-rubella (MMR) vaccine causes autism by damaging the lining of the intestines.

2. Thimerosal, a mercury-containing preservative in some vaccines, causes autism by damaging the nervous system.

3. Receiving too many vaccines at once leads to autism by affecting the immune system.

At this writing, there have been 29 studies since 1998 that have looked at the MMR vaccine and ASDs, and all have come to the same conclusion: there is no evidence that the MMR vaccine causes autism. For example, one study compared all children in Denmark (535,544) who got the MMR vaccine with children who didn't get the vaccine and found that the risk for ASDs was no different for children who received the MMR vaccine than for those children who did not.

Thimerosal is an organic mercury-containing antibacterial compound that was in US vaccines until 1999. There have been 11 studies since 1998 that have looked at thimerosal and ASDs, and all have come to the same conclusion: there is no evidence that children who received vaccines with thimerosal have a greater risk of autism than those who didn't. For example, a recent study comparing 200 children with ASDs with 700 children without ASDs showed that there were no differences in the amount of thimerosal that each group received from vaccines. Another study showed that groups of school-aged children exposed to smaller or larger amounts of thimerosal performed similarly on a series of psychologic tests. In addition, the rate that ASDs are diagnosed has continued to rise even though thimerosal has been removed from almost all vaccines for more than 10 years.

These days, a common concern is that getting a number of vaccines at the same time might somehow weaken the immune system, triggering the development of ASDs. Because of this belief, some have suggested that parents should space out vaccines by using an alternative vaccine schedule. There are a number of reasons why this is not recommended. First, receiving multiple vaccines at the same time is safe. Today's more refined vaccines even when given together cause *less* stress to the immune system than vaccines of the past. This means that even though children receive more vaccines at the same time, the challenge to the immune system is less than in years past. Secondly, there is evidence that delaying vaccines does not make a difference in development. A recent study comparing school-aged children who received their vaccines on time with those who did not found that timely vaccination was associated with better performance on numerous tests of language and intelligence. Less-vaccinated children did not do better on any of the tests. For parents who are concerned that children receive too many vaccines too soon or who believe delaying immunizations is beneficial, this study provides reassurance that timely vaccination during infancy has no adverse effect on long-term neuropsychologic outcomes. Lastly, it's important to understand that the vaccination schedule created by the CDC was designed to protect children when they are most vulnerable to disease. Delaying vaccines or not vaccinating your child puts him at risk for vaccine-preventable diseases. Even those who are fully vaccinated increase their chances of contracting a vaccine-preventable disease if they live in a community where many people are under-immunized. One study found that for every 1% increase in proportion of school-aged children who were under-immunized, the risk of pertussis infection among fully vaccinated children doubled.

Skipping or delaying vaccines also increases the risk for other children in your neighborhood. For example, many communities in the United States are currently experiencing outbreaks of measles because there are too many unvaccinated children. And unvaccinated children help the virus move more easily from person to person. If you have concerns about vaccines, be sure to talk with your child's pediatrician.

As of this writing, more than 40 studies since 1998 have been published in peer-reviewed literature, and all have come to the same conclusion: vaccines do not cause autism. Approximately 1% of the population has the condition, yet researchers all over the globe have examined the records of hundreds of thousands of children and could not find any evidence of a relationship between vaccines and autism. With such a large number of children studied, if there were a link between ASDs and vaccines, it would have shown up in one of these studies. For a listing of studies, visit www.HealthyChildren.org/vaccinestudies.

What scientists do know is that ASDs may often result from complex interactions between environmental exposures and a person's genes. So while you may be born with a genetic predisposition for ASDs, it requires an environmental exposure or event—which may even occur in the womb—for that gene to be expressed.

Some experts suspect that chemicals in our environment are involved in causing ASDs. Toxins like inorganic mercury have been touted as likely suspects, as have many other heavy metals, pesticides, and substances in plastics. The human-created class of chemicals known as polychlorinated biphenyls is also suspected as a culprit. But so far, there has not been enough research to prove these suspicions.

Experts do know that exposure to certain drugs during pregnancy can contribute to the development of ASDs. Two drugs in particular deserve mention. One of them is valproate, an anticonvulsant used to treat bipolar disorder and epilepsy. The other is thalidomide, a drug now used to treat multiple myeloma, a type of bone marrow and blood cancer. Thalidomide had been used to treat morning sickness in pregnant women in the late 1950s and early 1960s but was subsequently banned for causing birth defects. These medications are believed to affect the development of the fetus' brain in the early trimesters of pregnancy, a time when developmental abnormalities in the brain are most likely to occur.

Infections are often cited as a probable culprit too. But so far, only one infection—rubella—has been associated with autism. Rubella, also known as German measles, causes a rash, fever, and muscle and joint pain. Congenital rubella develops in a fetus when a mother is exposed to the rubella virus early in her pregnancy. Babies born with this disorder often have many birth defects in addition to severe developmental delays. They may also have symptoms of ASDs. In recent years, the disorder has become less of a concern since the rubella vaccine was introduced, which is ironically a component of the controversial MMR vaccine.

Recent studies suggest that babies exposed to large amounts of alcohol in the womb can develop ASDs as well as a spectrum of other neurodevelopmental disorders. These babies have fetal alcohol syndrome or alcohol-related neurodevelopmental disorder. They often have growth deficiencies that lead to short stature, small head circumference, decreased muscle tone, facial abnormalities, cardiac defects, and delayed development. Children with fetal alcohol syndrome may be also diagnosed with ASDs, though the link between autism and prenatal exposure to alcohol requires further research.

Family Health and History

The health of mom and dad always plays a major role in a child's health, so it's no surprise that experts have probed for links between family health and ASDs. In particular, scientists have zeroed in on the mother's history of autoimmune diseases, illnesses in which the body's immune system attacks itself. In particular, research has shown that children whose mothers have rheumatoid arthritis or celiac disease are more likely to have ASDs. Rheumatoid arthritis is a disease in which the body attacks the lining of the joints, causing inflammation and pain. In celiac disease, the body cannot tolerate gluten, a protein in wheat, rye, and barley. When someone with celiac disease eats gluten, the immune system launches an attack on the villi, small protrusions that line the small intestine.

The risk for an ASD also goes up if there is a family history of type 1 diabetes, another autoimmune illness. In people with type 1 diabetes, the immune system attacks cells in the pancreas and destroys its ability to make insulin, a hormone that's essential for turning the foods we eat, particularly carbohydrates, into energy. So while autism is not an autoimmune disorder, it's possible that the genes involved in causing autoimmune disease may also be playing a role in the development of ASDs. In women with rheumatoid arthritis, there is evidence that they may produce antibodies during pregnancy that affect fetal brain development.

Another factor in early pregnancy that appears to increase the risk for ASDs is advanced maternal and paternal age. Studies have shown that older parents were more likely to have a child with an ASD than younger parents. One study found that for mothers aged 20 to 39 years, every 10-year increase in their age raised the risk of them having a child with an ASD by 38%.

No one knows exactly why older women and men are more likely to have children with an ASD, but experts suspect that a woman's hormonal changes at an older age could affect fetal brain development. In addition, they suspect that the use of reproductive technologies may play a role. Simply being older causes more age-related changes in a woman's genes and adds to the cumulative effects of exposures to environmental toxins, both of which may affect the fetus. Older men have a great number of spontaneous genetic mutations in their sperm as they age, which may contribute to higher risk for an ASD. But more research is needed to know exactly how advanced parental age affects risk for ASDs.

PREGNANCY COMPLICATIONS AND BABY'S HEALTH AT BIRTH MAY AFFECT RISK FOR AUTISM SPECTRUM DISORDERS

Data from several studies published in 2009 indicated that mothers who have gestational diabetes are more likely to have babies with autism spectrum disorders (ASDs). Gestational diabetes occurs when pregnant women develop high blood sugar. The condition is usually detected with an oral glucose tolerance test in the 24th to 28th week of pregnancy. Glucose levels usually return to normal after delivery.

In fact, a number of prenatal and perinatal risk factors are associated with ASDs. Some of these include premature birth, fetal distress, low birth weight, and birth trauma. But just because there is an association does not mean that these factors *cause* ASDs. These are just conditions that may elevate risk.

A baby born with encephalopathy, for example, has an elevated risk of developing an ASD. Encephalopathy is a term used to describe any type of brain disease that alters the brain's function or structure. One study showed that 5% of survivors of newborn encephalopathy were later diagnosed with an ASD. It's possible that these children were genetically predisposed to encephalopathy or an ASD.

In addition, babies who are jaundiced at birth may be more likely to develop an ASD. Jaundice is the yellow color seen in the skin of many newborns. It occurs when a newborn's liver can't break down bilirubin, a substance in bile produced by the breakdown of red blood cells. A study found that babies who had jaundice were at greater risk for ASDs, especially if they were born to mothers who previously had children and if they were born between October and March. While the study does not say that jaundice causes autism, it does suggest that jaundice may be among the factors that elevate risk.

The amount of time between pregnancies—also known as the inter-pregnancy interval—is also a risk factor. One study that examined birth records of second-born children found that those who were conceived within 12 months of the birth of their older sibling were more than 3 times more likely to be diagnosed with ASDs. Children conceived 12 to 23 months after an older sibling were almost 2 times more likely to have been diagnosed with ASDs.

Ongoing Research

Solving the mystery of what causes ASDs has spawned intense research efforts around the world. Some of the major research projects now underway are

- The Centers for Autism and Developmental Disabilities Research and Epidemiology is being directed by the CDC in California, Colorado, Maryland, North Carolina, Pennsylvania, and Georgia. Each center is working on aspects of a project called Study to Explore Early Development and looking for causes and risk factors of ASDs. In California, for instance, the focus is on identifying biological traits that will help with early identification of children with ASDs and in investigating potential environmental risk factors. For more information, see www.cdc.gov/ncbddd/autism/caddre.html.

- Early Autism Risk Longitudinal Investigation (EARLI) is following more than 1,200 mothers from pregnancy through the first 3 years of their babies' lives to examine potential environmental risk factors that may be involved in ASDs. The EARLI study will look at the DNA profiles of all family members and test the hypothesis that ASDs have a genetic and an epigenetic basis. Research is being done at multiple sites including Johns Hopkins, Drexel University, Children's Hospital of Philadelphia/University of Pennsylvania, and Kaiser Permanente in northern California. For more information, see www.earlistudy.org.

- The Centers for Children's Environmental Health and Disease Prevention (CCEHDP), which is supported by the National Institute of Environmental Health Sciences and Environmental Protection Agency, is examining the effect of exposure to chemicals such as lead, mercury, and pesticides on neurodevelopmental disorders such as ASDs, attention-deficit/hyperactivity disorder, and developmental delays. The research is being done at several sites including the University of California, Davis (UC Davis), and the University of Medicine & Dentistry of New Jersey. For more information, see www.niehs. nih.gov/research/supported/centers/prevention.

- At UC Davis, the CCEHDP has established the first large epidemiologic study of ASDs called Childhood Autism Risks from Genetics and the Environment. This study, which is also being conducted at the University of California, Los Angeles, will involve up to 2,000 children with ASDs and other developmental delays or intellectual disabilities as well as children with typical or expected development. It will examine various aspects of their lives before and after birth, such as environmental exposures, medical history, and diet, as well as physiologic factors that may affect brain development such as specific genes, lipids like cholesterol, and molecules involved in the immune and nervous systems. The study will involve children born in California who are between the ages of 24 and 54 months.

- The National Children's Study is examining the effects of genetics and the environment— including air, water, and diet, as well as cultural and community influences and family dynamics—on the health of children across the country, from birth to age 21 years. The study also involves pregnant women and women who may become pregnant. Findings will be used to help improve the health of children. For more information, see www.nationalchildrensstudy.gov.

Understanding the causes of ASDs is critical to improving prognosis for children diagnosed with this disorder. It will also pave the way to more effective treatments. Ultimately, knowing the cause of ASDs may even help us find ways to prevent this baffling disorder.

> **I have a daughter who has an autism spectrum disorder (ASD) and a son who does not. Could my son carry a gene for ASDs that he'll pass on to his offspring?**
>
> Experts know that if one child in the family has an ASD, that child's siblings are at greater risk for developing ASDs too. If your son is healthy, the odds that he will pass on a gene for ASDs is low. However, his odds may be slightly higher than someone else who does not have a sibling with an ASD. The genetics underlying ASDs are complex, and it may be helpful for parents to seek counseling from a geneticist or genetic counselor to better understand the risk of recurrence.

Autism Champion: Alison Singer

Alison Singer was a successful television executive at NBC when her daughter Jodie was diagnosed with autism in 2000. The diagnosis changed Alison's life forever. She left television and became acting CEO of Autism Speaks when it was launched in 2005.

In 2009, she founded her own organization, the Autism Science Foundation. The group raises money to support ASD research, brings together parents and scientists to share information, and trains scientists to work with the media. It also brings the latest science to people at the forefront of ASD—parents and educators.

Getting the science out is Alison's way of combating the myths that continue to linger about vaccines and the unproven remedies that are often touted as treatments. Even now, Alison gets frequent e-mails offering an alleged cure. "These quacks prey on the desperation of parents who are willing to try anything they think might possibly help their child," she says. "Believe me, I get it. We love our children so much and want them to improve and so we are willing to try anything. That's why it's so important to do the science to test interventions. We need to know what works and what doesn't. These are not quick fixes; they take time and lots of effort, but they really do help."

Jodie is now 14 years old. Time has taught Alison that with the right therapies, children with ASDs can make significant improvement. "The day they're diagnosed is the bottom," says Alison, who also has a younger daughter who does not have an ASD. "It's the worst day. From then on, the kids will continue to gain skills. They will make gains that astonish you, even if it's sometimes 2 steps forward and 1 step back. Those steps back are frustrating, but I have learned to appreciate the steps forward more than I ever imagined was possible."

Her advice to parents? Talk to other parents in your community. "Services are always delivered locally," she says. "Your best source of information will often be other parents in your school district."

CHAPTER 3

How Do I Know if
My Child Has an
Autism Spectrum Disorder?

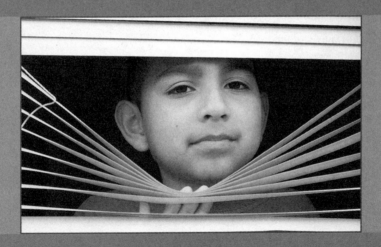

Carly was concerned. At 17 months, her son Asher wasn't talking yet, and when she called his name, he would rarely respond. At the 18-month visit, Asher's pediatrician listened to her concerns and performed an autism screening test. He informed her that he also shared her concerns about Asher's behavior and development. Asher was referred to a specialty clinic and subsequently diagnosed with an autism spectrum disorder (ASD). While the diagnosis was a shock to his family, they were ultimately thankful to have their concerns validated. The diagnostic evaluation also allowed them to learn more about Asher and how to help him. Today, at the age of 7, Asher still faces challenges with social skills and communication but is making steady progress, much to the delight of his family.

≈ ≈ ≈ ≈ ≈

Getting a diagnosis for a child with an ASD often isn't easy. Unlike some conditions, such as diabetes or celiac disease, ASDs aren't diagnosed with a blood test. There are currently no x-rays or scans that can detect ASDs. Instead, diagnosis is made based on caregivers' description of the child's development and by careful observations of characteristic behaviors by providers who have expertise with ASDs. In some cases, the path to a diagnosis begins with something as simple as a parent's hunch or a sense that something isn't quite right.

Diagnosing an ASD is difficult for many reasons. For one, every single case is different. While children on the autism spectrum share similar characteristics, exactly how those traits play out will vary from one child to the next. The severity of autism varies considerably too. For example, some people with ASDs have very mild forms, display virtually no speech problems, and are capable of independently meeting their needs as adults. Some may even be considered gifted and exceptionally bright. Others have severe forms of the disorder, with significant disability, and may have a lifelong dependence on others to meet their needs. Still others have genetic disorders or medically complex conditions requiring medical stabilization before a child's developmental status can be accurately determined.

One thing experts do know now is that early diagnosis and treatment of an ASD is very important in determining how well a child lives with it. Herein lies the challenge. While most signs of ASDs are apparent by the time a child is 3 years old, many children are not diagnosed until they are older.

Age of diagnosis may depend on where children fall on the spectrum as well as other socio-economic factors. One study found that the average age of diagnosis in children with ASDs was 3.1 years, while those with pervasive development disorder–not otherwise specified (PDD-NOS) was 3.9 years. Among children with Asperger syndrome, the average age of diagnosis was 7.2 years. The study also uncovered some possible explanations as to why some children are diagnosed sooner and others are diagnosed later. Children were typically diagnosed later if they lived in a rural setting, came from households with lower incomes, and had consulted 4 or more different primary care physicians. Symptoms make a difference too; children who had severe language delays were diagnosed an average of 1.2 years earlier than those who did not. Those who demonstrated hand flapping, toe walking, and unusual play over a period were diagnosed at a younger age, while those who were oversensitive to pain or had a hearing impairment tended to be diagnosed later.

Children with ASDs who have intellectual disabilities (or global developmental delays) are usually diagnosed earlier than those who do not. Those who have regressive autism, in which signs of ASDs appear after a period of seemingly normal development, are also more likely to be diagnosed early. Boys are generally diagnosed at a younger age than girls. It's possible that certain traits in girls with ASDs, such as shyness, may be more socially acceptable and therefore more easily overlooked.

Although diagnosing a child at a young age is important for getting the early intervention that is so critical to children with ASDs, a national study has shown that the median age of diagnosis was 6 years, and more than a quarter of children were not diagnosed until age 8. The good news is that the age of earliest diagnosed cases is dropping. According to the Centers for Disease Control and Prevention (CDC), the earliest cases were diagnosed between 49 and 66 months in 2002; by 2006, earliest cases were diagnosed between 41 and 60 months of age; and by 2008, the age of earliest case identification was between 36 and 59 months.

Early diagnosis requires a partnership between parents and pediatricians. Within this partnership you, as the parent, should feel comfortable bringing up any concerns you have about your child's behavior or development—the way she plays, learns, speaks, and acts. Likewise, your child's pediatrician's role in the partnership is to listen and act on your concerns. During your child's visits, the pediatrician may ask specific questions or complete a questionnaire about your child's development. Pediatricians take these steps because they understand the value of early diagnosis and intervention and know where to refer you if concerns are identified. This chapter will help you recognize the early signs of ASDs so that you can better partner with your child's pediatrician to get your child the help she needs. The importance of this partnership cannot be stressed enough.

Begin Early in Infancy

Like adults, all babies are unique. Some start babbling early on, while others are late talkers. Some start crawling at a young age; others seem to take longer to start moving about. Even within families, parents often marvel at how differently their children grow and develop. But experts are increasingly convinced that early signs of ASDs are evident even during the first few years of life.

While it may be challenging to diagnose an ASD in a child younger than 2 years, it is important for you as a parent to monitor your child's development carefully so that you can identify any concerns as soon as possible. For instance, by the end of their third month, most babies have started to smile and show pleasure in playing with others and are gradually becoming more communicative with their expressions and body movement. They're usually able to raise their head and chest when they're on their tummies and stretch out their legs and kick. Place their tiny feet on a firm surface and they will push down. Most can open and shut their hands and bring their hand to their mouth. They usually can reach for dangling objects and are starting to take hold of toys.

Meanwhile, they may be watching you intently and following moving objects. They can often recognize familiar objects and people from a distance. They may smile at the sound of your voice and turn their heads in the direction of sound. Some may be cooing (making vowel sounds) and imitating the sounds you make.

In babies who may have developmental disabilities such as ASDs, some of these milestones may be delayed or absent. Babies with ASDs may only rarely respond to loud noises, smile at others, or reach for objects. Some may seldom take note of their hands or follow moving objects. They may only occasionally vocalize, pay attention to new faces, or support their head well.

Of course, even perfectly healthy babies may not achieve these milestones by the end of 3 months of age either. Some babies simply develop a little more slowly. If your baby does not meet all of these milestones on time, it does not necessarily mean she has an ASD or another developmental disability. While ASDs and other developmental disabilities are not typically diagnosed during infancy, children who are late achieving developmental milestones benefit from treatment. If your child does display signs of a developmental delay, you can contact an early intervention or Part C services program, which is geared to help infants and toddlers from birth through age 3 who may be at risk for a developmental disorder. We'll discuss those in greater detail in Chapter 5. Most important of all, watching for these signs will make you aware of a potential problem, so you can bring it to your pediatrician's attention. If these delays persist or new ones develop, you and your child's pediatrician can intervene at an earlier age to help your child reach her full potential.

What to Look for in Autism Spectrum Disorders

When your child has a cold, you expect a runny nose, some coughing, and perhaps a low-grade fever. When your child has eczema, you know his skin will itch and develop a rash. But when your child has an ASD, it's a lot harder to know what to expect, especially given how different the condition reveals itself in each child. But there are some major characteristics that are common to most children with ASDs.

Unusual Language Development

Language development varies widely among children with ASDs. Some are early talkers and never seem to run out of things to say. Others are naturally quiet and start speaking much later. Speech typically begins with producing vowel sounds, or cooing, in the first few months of life. By 6 months of age babies can combine consonants and vowels, called babbling, making simple sounds like "da" or "ba." Babbling gradually evolves as your baby starts to link these sounds ("da da") and introduce new ones such as "pa."

Between 4 and 6 months the typically developing child will display a back-and-forth pattern of speaking that alternates between cooing or babbling and silence. For instance, babies often vocalize to themselves when they first wake up, only to fall silent when mom enters the room, as if waiting to hear what she has to say. When mom leaves to retrieve diapers, they may start vocalizing again. When babies vocalize in this manner, it is possible for caregivers to sustain a "conversation" with them in which turn-taking occurs, adults speaking in regular sentences and babies cooing and babbling. These back-and-forth vocalizations, together with eye contact and shared emotions (elements of nonverbal or body language), set the stage for later conversations using real words. Over time, a baby's sounds become more distinct and start to sound like words. Eventually, the typical child will begin to form short sentences.

Most parents are eager to hear their children utter their first words. A child's first utterances often inspire awe and excitement. So it's not surprising that when these events do not occur, parents are apt to take notice and bring it up with their child's pediatrician. Language delays are often the first signs noticed by parents and doctors that raise concern that a child may have an ASD. They're often the first indication to a pediatrician that a child needs evaluation.

Language differences characterize all forms of ASDs, to varying degrees. In some children with ASDs, language skills may be absent or delayed. Other children, like those diagnosed with Asperger syndrome, may possess advanced speaking skills but struggle having a back-and-forth conversation because they have the need to speak only about a preferred topic. This type of language challenge common to children with Asperger syndrome reflects qualitative differences in language development that distinguish their language skills from those of typically developing peers. Specifically, these differences are in the area of pragmatic language—using language for social communication.

Pragmatic language involves skills such as picking up on body language, maintaining eye contact, understanding implied meaning, using normal voice inflection and volume when speaking, maintaining the topic of conversation, and recognizing the interest level of others in what is being discussed. Such differences may not be obvious until preschool when interacting with peers. Whereas many children with ASDs have language delays, such as those with autistic disorder and PDD-NOS, all children on the autism spectrum have challenges with pragmatic language.

Most language delays are evident by the time a child is 18 months old. It is most apparent if you notice that your child is not showing the desire to communicate or express himself with gestures such as pointing. Children who have milder forms of autism will usually develop speech, but their language may be odd and lack purpose. For example, they may say words that seem to have no intent and that may be taken from television programs or movies. The early speech patterns of children with ASDs may have some distinctly unusual patterns.

Echolalia

Echolalia is the repetition of another person's speech. It may be *immediate,* meaning the child will repeat what he hears right after he hears it, or *delayed,* meaning the repeated phrase will pop up hours, days, or even weeks later.

Keep in mind, though, that echolalia can occur in children who do not have ASDs too. The difference, however, is that in children who do not have ASDs, echolalia tends to be of the immediate kind and then completely disappears from the child's vocabulary. In children who have ASDs, echolalia may last throughout their lives. And the degree of echolalia significantly affects their ability to communicate effectively with others.

They also tend to display a mix of immediate and delayed echolalia and are more likely to repeat larger chunks of material. For example, rather than repeat the slogan of a television commercial, they may recite the entire commercial and do so for long periods, even while others are trying to communicate with them.

At first, echolalia may create the impression that a child with an ASD is verbally gifted. His vocabulary, grammar, and syntax may make him sound sophisticated for his age. Some kids may even display remarkable skills at labeling colors, shapes, letters, and numbers. But in the child with an ASD, the voice may be delivered in a monotone fashion or other type of peculiar intonation. A closer listen often reveals delayed or absent receptive language, which means difficulty understanding what is spoken to him. Most children with typical development are able to follow simple one-step commands by the time they are 12 to 15 months old. If you ask a child with an ASD to get a toy, he is less likely to respond. If you ask him to identify a familiar object, such as a sippy cup or shoe, from amongst several items, he is often unable.

Pop-up Words

Some children with ASDs will say a word without any provocation and seemingly no reason. Delivery is entirely spontaneous and often inconsistent. For instance, a child may be playing with a ball when he starts saying "Dog," when there is no dog—real, stuffed, or in pictures—nearby, nor has a dog been recently seen. In some children, the pop-up word will be spoken during times of stress, such as the child in the dentist's office who says "Bye-bye" when the dentist attempts to place him in the procedure chair. Pop-up words can last for days or weeks and then disappear.

Giant Words

Children with ASDs sometimes say phrases that link together several words, such as "Whatisit? Idontknow." These phrases are spoken without true meaning, and the children are unable to combine words into sentences that have any real meaning.

Some children appear to master all the language skills appropriate for their age, only to have them diminish between 15 and 24 months of age, often at 18 to 21 months. These children may have regressive autism. When a child has regression, he may lose verbal skills as well as communicative gestures. The loss may be sudden or gradual. For many parents, the loss of language skills is often a red flag that something is amiss.

For more information about how your infant and young toddler should be communicating with you, see "Milestones During the First 2 Years" on page 48.

Social Skill Deficits

Human beings are hardwired for socializing. We want to share our lives with other people, so we gather for meals, throw parties, and meet for coffee. The drive to be social starts in infancy when babies gaze adoringly at their parents, coo at the sound of their voices, and later point at objects they want to see. In children with ASDs, that desire for connectedness is diminished or absent. Children with ASDs may be content to be left alone and are less likely to seek out others for interaction. The lack of social reciprocity may seem to emerge in toddlerhood, but experts now know that more basic social skill deficits can be apparent even

MILESTONES DURING THE FIRST 2 YEARS

Long before your baby utters her first word, she has already started communicating with you, using smiles, looks, movements, and sounds. Children develop at different rates, but they usually are able to do certain things at certain ages. Following are general developmental milestones. Keep in mind that they are only guidelines. If you have *any* questions about your baby's development, ask your child's pediatrician—the sooner the better. Even when there are delays, early intervention can make a significant difference.

By 1 year, most babies will

- Look for and be able to find where a sound is coming from.
- Respond to their name most of the time when you call it.
- Wave goodbye.
- Look where you point when you say, "Look at the _____."
- Babble with intonation (voice rises and falls as if they are speaking in sentences).
- Take turns "talking" with you—listen and pay attention to you when you speak and then resume babbling when you stop.
- Say "da-da" to dad and "ma-ma" to mom.
- Say at least 1 word.
- Point to items they want that are out of reach or make sounds while pointing.

Between 1 and 2 years, most toddlers will

- Follow simple commands, first when the adult speaks and gestures, and then later with words alone.
- Get objects from another room when asked.
- Point to a few body parts when asked.
- Point to interesting objects or events to get you to look at them too.
- Bring things to you to show you.
- Point to objects so you will name them.
- Name a few common objects and pictures when asked.
- Enjoy pretending (for example, pretend cooking). They will use gestures and words with you or with a favorite stuffed animal or doll.
- Learn about 1 new word per week between 1½ and 2 years.

MILESTONES DURING THE FIRST 2 YEARS, CONTINUED

By 2 years of age, most toddlers will

- Point to many body parts and common objects.
- Point to some pictures in books.
- Follow 1-step commands without a gesture like "Put your cup on the table."
- Be able to say about 50 to 100 words.
- Say several 2-word sentences and phrases like "Daddy go," "Doll mine," and "All gone."
- Be understood by others (or by adults) about half of the time.

---

earlier. Crucial building blocks of more advanced social skills include joint attention, social orienting, and pretend play.

Joint Attention

A toddler does not look at Elmo on the television despite his father's pointing and saying, "Look!" A young child finishes a drawing of his mother but does not bring it over to show her. A school-aged child rarely shares what happens at school with his parents despite their repeated requests. These children with ASDs all demonstrate deficits in joint attention. Joint attention is engaging another's attention to objects, events, or other persons simply for the enjoyment of sharing an experience. Like all developmental milestones, it is mastered in steps that occur at predictable ages throughout childhood.

Joint attention starts early when a typically developing baby recognizes a parent or familiar caregiver's voice, smiles, and reacts with happy smiles of his own. At about 8 months of age, the baby will follow your gaze when it shifts away to see what you are looking at. Sometime between 10 and 12 months of age, when you point in the direction of an interesting object or event and say, "Look!" your baby will respond by turning his head to see what's intriguing you. Your baby will then turn his gaze back to you to affirm that he saw what you were indicating.

In children who have ASDs, this type of experience sharing may not develop at the same rate. Babies with ASDs are less likely to look in your direction or show interest in engaging you. Saying the baby's name loudly or touching him on the shoulder may not get his attention. Even if it does, a child with an ASD is not as likely to look back at you to share in what you've both just looked at.

The difficulty with social engagement continues into toddlerhood. At about 12 months, the typically developing child will begin trying to assert himself socially by asking for an object that is out of reach. He may do this by making simple sounds like "uh" or pointing with an index finger. This is called imperative pointing, or pointing to request. By about 14 to 16 months of age, the child with typical development will point at objects he likes simply to comment to you that it is pleasing to him and to share that experience with you. This is called declarative pointing, or pointing to show. He will alternate between looking at you and at the object or event that has captured his interest. This is the full expression of joint attention. Consistently demonstrating joint attention, experts say, reliably predicts whether a child will develop functional language within a year.

Delayed or lack of joint attention is one of the most specific early signs of ASD. Compared to children with typical development, children with ASDs are less likely to point to or comment about objects or events. When they do point, they may show little enthusiasm and make little effort to connect with you while pointing. Although some children with ASDs may point to shapes, objects, and colors they have learned, it is more often to label than to share an experience. Despite these challenges, numerous studies have shown that with early intervention, children with ASDs can improve their joint attention.

Social Orienting

The first time a baby turns her head at the sound of her name is an exciting moment for most parents. Developmentally, it's also an important social skill milestone, known as social orienting. This milestone is usually achieved by the time a child is 8 to 10 months old.

Children who have ASDs may not acknowledge a caregiver's bid for their attention. It may take calling a child's name louder and louder to finally get her attention. Failure to respond to their name is one of the most common early signs of ASD in young children but is sometimes overlooked. While it is important to consider the possibility of a hearing problem, most children with ASDs hear and respond to environmental sounds (for example, the doorbell) but seem to respond less to the human voice. With time and intervention, most children with ASDs will improve their ability to respond to their name.

Pretend Play Skills and Friendships

As you might imagine, you will notice differences in the way children with ASDs play with toys and with other children. Typically developing children will begin playing by grasping objects, a skill that develops around 4 months of age. They may start mouthing objects, and at 8 to 10 months of age may start banging toys together or against the floor or table, or tossing them around. This stage of play is known as the sensory-motor stage. Around 1 year, they become more aware of how toys are meant to be handled and may start playing with them more appropriately. For instance, instead of banging blocks on the floor, they may now stack the blocks. Soon after, pretend play emerges, and they may use toy bottles to feed a baby doll or a toy telephone to chat with grandma. Pretend play gradually becomes more sophisticated, and simple objects may be used to represent other, more complex ones. Bananas, for instance, may become telephones, and wooden blocks may be used as cars.

Compared with typical children, children with ASDs engage in significantly less pretend play before the age of 2. They may have very little interest in toys, preferring instead to play with everyday objects like string, pens, and rocks. If they do develop an interest in toys, they may tend to play with parts of the toy and not the whole toy itself. So rather than push a toy truck along the floor, a boy with an ASD might pick it up and focus on spinning the wheels or opening and closing the doors. Children with ASDs who have normal nonverbal intelligence may be especially skilled at putting things together, such as stacking cups and assembling puzzles, and may later on become masterful at computer games, or what is called constructive play. Some children with ASDs may also insist on repeatedly lining up objects, which is known as ritualistic play. These types of play do not involve imitation, observation, or other people and are better suited for children who do better at play that involves trial and error problem-solving skills.

What can be deceiving is that some children with ASDs enjoy roughhousing. They may like it when dad tosses them in the air or tickles them on the floor. Many children who have ASDs enjoy the sensory-motor aspects of this type of play. Though it may appear to be "typical" behavior, it is often the sensory aspect of this kind of play that a child with an ASD prefers as opposed to the social engagement. In other words, they are seeking out the sensory stimulation that occurs when they are tossed or tickled, not necessarily the companionship of the other person.

To the unsuspecting parent, a child with an ASD may appear easy to manage because he is content to play by himself for hours without seeking out mom or dad. But a closer look at the child's style of play will reveal that the play is sensory-motor, constructive, and ritualistic, and does not involve other people. Later on in life, the child with an ASD often struggles to interact with peers and cooperate in groups with social rules. As a result, children with ASDs are often the victims of bullying and left out of most social circles.

Repetitive and Unusual Behaviors

Children who have ASDs may display different behaviors and peculiar mannerisms. They may flap their hands, rock their bodies, or twirl their fingers, especially when they become excited. Some children walk on their toes, nod their heads, or sniff and lick nonfood items. These behaviors are called stereotypies, repetitive behaviors that outwardly serve no apparent purpose and yet are performed compulsively. Stereotypies are generally harmless but can, in some cases, interfere with the child doing something else or prevent the child from learning a new skill. Stereotypies may not be obvious until after the age of 2.

Although stereotypies are common in children with ASDs, they don't just occur with autism. Children who have intellectual disabilities or global developmental delays may also demonstrate stereotypies. Even young children with typical development may sometimes flap their hands when they're excited or go through periods of walking on their toes.

Restricted Interests

Most children don't escape childhood without developing a strong bond to a beloved teddy bear, special blanket, or treasured doll. Children with ASDs, on the other hand, may not, preferring instead to latch on to a hard object such as a pen, a flashlight, or an action figure.

The attachment to that object is also more persistent, and they may insist more intensely on holding the object at all times.

Children who have Asperger syndrome may be less consumed with objects and more enamored with topics and facts. But the fierce interest in these topics is often stronger than it is in children with typical development. In some cases, the child with Asperger syndrome may have an encyclopedic storehouse of facts and information about the topic. Topics of interest are not necessarily unusual for small children. For instance, Ellen's son Brian developed a strong interest in dinosaurs, which was no surprise because his father is a paleo-artist who has several paleontologists as friends. Besides, many young children are fascinated with dinosaurs. But Brian's interest in dinosaurs has been all-consuming. He is often more than willing to discuss dinosaurs with others, to the exclusion of other subjects, even when his classmates show no interest. The intensity of his interest is common in children who have Asperger syndrome.

Other Common Features of Autism Spectrum Disorders

Language differences and deficits in social skills are the most prominent and defining characteristics of children with ASDs. But many children also have other difficulties.

Cognitive Challenges

Although cognitive deficits aren't considered a core feature of ASDs, they are common among children who have these disorders. At one time, experts estimated that intellectual disability—the term varies depending on age and different assessment tools—applied to 90% of all children with an ASD. The latest data from the CDC indicate that these problems affect about 38% of children with ASDs. As you may recall, children who have Asperger syndrome do not have cognitive disabilities and have normal, or even above-normal, intellectual skills.

What many children with ASDs do have is unevenness in their skills and development. A child with an ASD may, for instance, be an exceptional math whiz but may struggle to read. Some children may also have incredible focus, memory, and mathematic skills, while others display notable musical and artistic talents. In rare instances, the child with an ASD may have highly developed skills and talents that earn him the label of savant. A savant—as performed by Dustin Hoffman in the movie *Rain Man*—is a person with exceptional skills in a narrow area. For example, some savants may be capable of doing rapid calculations, memorizing large amounts of information, and mastering complex pieces of music with little practice. Savant abilities are somewhat rare (ranging from less than 1% up to 10%) in children and adults with ASDs.

Sensory-Motor Symptoms

For children with ASDs, the sounds, sights, and textures that we experience on a daily basis can often be a challenging minefield to navigate. Some are hypersensitive, or overly bothered, by things in their environment. Others are hyposensitive and completely insensitive to sensations that others consider bothersome. But a child's sensitivity to sights and sounds may not be consistent across the senses. For example, loud noises at a party may put a child with an ASD on edge, even though she's totally oblivious to the sound of her mother's voice calling her name. A child with an ASD might excessively inspect toys or other objects by gazing at them for a particularly long time or from different angles, while remaining uninterested in the rest of her surroundings.

Some children have tactile defensiveness, in which they're overly sensitive to certain textures and surfaces, like the elastic in socks or labels in shirts. Some may resist hugs because they don't like to be touched. They may also have oral aversions to certain textures in food. Children with ASDs may also show unusual sensory-seeking behaviors, such as a tendency to walk on their toes (even though they have full range of motion at their ankles), flap their hands, spin, rock back and forth, jump, or chew on objects.

Some children with ASDs have unusual motor skills. Some may appear to have advanced fine motor skills such as stringing beads, but most have trouble with gross motor skills like running, climbing, and jumping. Many also have trouble with coordination and motor planning, which involve thinking through a task and then doing the movements in the proper sequence. Children with Asperger syndrome, in particular, may be clumsy. Some children may appear hyperactive and show symptoms of attention-deficit/hyperactivity disorder (ADHD). Others may be withdrawn and hypoactive, and make little movement.

Common Health Problems

Children with ASDs often have other health and psychiatric conditions. These associated conditions may have profound effects on them. They can often affect children's behavior, their ability to learn, and their overall health and well-being. Treating these conditions may help a child's overall functioning, which is why talking to your child's pediatrician about them is critical. In fact, a child may have one or several of these problems. Medications to help control some of these conditions will be discussed in Chapter 6. Here are some common problems in children with ASDs.

Seizures and Epilepsy

Children with ASDs are more likely than children with typical development to experience a seizure—sudden and excessive electrical discharges in the brain that can produce a variety of symptoms from unconsciousness and contractions of the muscles to undirected, uncontrolled, and unorganized movements. Seizures are more common in children with ASDs who have global developmental delay, intellectual disability, severe motor deficits, and a family history of epilepsy. During a seizure, a child may make jerky movements with his limbs, lose consciousness, or stare off into space. Seizures in children with ASDs are most common when the child is younger than 5 years and again during adolescence. Children with ASDs who are suspected to have seizures may require additional tests, including an electroencephalogram (EEG) or an imaging test of the brain, to confirm seizures and look for potential causes.

Gastrointestinal Disorders

Children with ASDs may be more likely to have gastrointestinal (GI) issues than typically developing children. Many children with ASDs experience chronic constipation, diarrhea, vomiting, and abdominal pain. Most GI disorders in children with or without ASDs are functional, meaning that there is not a specific cause within the GI tract that can be identified. This is especially true for some GI disorders such as constipation, which may be the result of a child's selective eating habits and pickiness about food. Some GI disorders have an organic cause, meaning that there is a specific problem in the GI tract causing symptoms. This is true for GI disorders such as celiac disease, an autoimmune condition triggered by gluten and related proteins. It is especially important to tell your child's pediatrician about any weight loss, GI bleeding, prolonged or persistent vomiting, prolonged diarrhea, abdominal pain that is only in a small area of the abdomen, or fever because these may be symptoms of a more serious organic GI disorder.

Children with GI issues and ASDs may have difficulty informing their caregivers that they have abdominal pain. Instead, you may notice behaviors such as frequent clearing of the throat, screaming, whining, groaning, and sobbing for no apparent reason. Some children may display delayed echolalia and repeat a phrase they've heard in the past about their stomach or pain, such as, "Does your tummy hurt?"

Other children may grimace, grit their teeth, or wince. Some may mouth their clothing, lean their abdomen against furniture, or tap their fingers on their throat. Some children may eat, drink, and swallow more. Unusual postures such as the arching of the back, self-injurious behaviors, or an increase in repetitive behaviors may also be signs of GI distress.

Abdominal pain or discomfort can result in changes in a child's overall well-being too. You may notice your child becomes irritable or may develop sleep problems. It is important to tell your child's pediatrician about these symptoms or any of the other nonverbal behaviors common with GI conditions. After listening to you and examining your child, the pediatrician might choose to try a medicine to treat the most likely GI disorder (like constipation or gastroesophageal reflux) or do further testing for some of these conditions.

While ongoing research is exploring whether some children with ASDs have unique problems within the GI tract, the current way to treat GI disorders in children with ASDs is the same as for children without ASDs. This is because it is assumed that the problems within the GI tract are the same for both sets of children. There is no evidence at this point that children with ASDs have unique microscopic abnormalities in their intestines or overgrowth of yeast or other organisms that worsen behavior.

As of this printing, there also is no evidence that GI problems directly cause ASDs. One such theory was put forward in the 1990s. It claimed that changes in the GI tract (a "leaky gut") caused by the measles-mumps-rubella vaccine given to 1-year-olds actually caused

ASDs. This study was later found to be significantly flawed and was retracted from the medical literature. Despite many theories of a GI basis for autism, there hasn't been any proof of a specific link between a disordered GI system and symptoms of ASDs. (See Chapter 7 for more information on this issue.)

Tics

Some children with ASDs have tics—brief, involuntary movements and sounds that are also the defining symptoms of a neurologic condition called Tourette syndrome. The 2 conditions have a lot in common, including echolalia, obsessive-compulsive behaviors, and abnormal motor behaviors. There is some evidence to suggest that some of the same brain abnormalities in ASDs also exist in Tourette syndrome. In moderate to severe cases, medical treatment can be quite helpful.

Sleep Disorders

Studies show that between 40% and 80% of children with an ASD experience sleep problems. They may have trouble falling asleep, staying asleep, or waking up early. Severe sleep problems may affect a child's quality of life, worsen his ability to pay attention, and cause him to be irritable and display more repetitive behaviors. Likewise, caregivers of children with sleep problems will likely have sleep interruptions as well, adding to a family's overall stress level. Some children with ASDs appear to need less sleep than their typical peers. It is important to discuss sleep problems with your child's pediatrician because they may be caused by other medical conditions (such as gastroesophageal reflux) that cause pain and lead to night awakenings. (See Chapter 6.)

Attention-deficit/hyperactivity Disorder

Many children with ASDs have difficulty staying on task and focusing and may be impulsive and hyperactive. Some children on the autism spectrum wind up being diagnosed with ADHD as well. Attention-deficit/hyperactivity disorder is a biological, brain-based condition that, left untreated, can lead to difficulties in school, low self-esteem, and problems making friends. The condition is quite common and affects an estimated 6% to 9% of all school-aged children.

Children with ADHD have trouble filtering out irrelevant information. They struggle with prioritizing, organizing, and delaying gratification. In children who have ASDs, however, inattention may be related to self-directed thoughts or activities, such as the persistent repetition of a word, gesture, or act, rather than to minor distractions in the environment.

Aggression and Self-injury

Many children with ASDs have difficulty moderating the intensity of their emotions and controlling their impulses. Combined with the frustration of not being able to easily communicate their wants and needs, children with ASDs may exhibit aggressive behaviors and self-injury. On the other hand, a painful ear infection may cause a child to bang her head against the wall. Acting aggressively may also stem from stomach cramps caused by constipation. Aggressive behavior may be caused by an underlying psychiatric condition such as anxiety. With so many different causes, if your child is becoming aggressive toward others or herself, you should talk to your child's pediatrician. Often it will be necessary for a number of professionals to work together to find out the cause of the aggression. Once the cause is known, there are many potential therapies that help.

Anxiety Disorders

Children with ASDs are prone to anxiety, which may show up as anything from feelings of nervousness to hyperactivity and other inappropriate behaviors such as screaming or aggressive acts. Because many children with ASDs are extremely rigid in their routines, unexpected changes can lead to an increase in anxiety and inappropriate behaviors. Anxiety may be more common in children whose families have a history of this condition. Children with ASDs who have challenges communicating may become anxious if they do not know how to respond or cope appropriately.

Children with ASDs who have anxiety can sometimes become obsessive in their behaviors. Many children become extremely rigid in their routines. They may want to move through their mornings in the exact same order every day and insist, for example, that their stuffed animals be laid out in the same precise arrangement every day. When those rituals and routines are disrupted, they may have trouble adapting or have more intense or prolonged tantrums when caregivers try to transition them from one activity to another.

Depression

Children who have ASDs are more vulnerable to depression, a mood disorder that in children with typical development may lead to sadness, inactivity, and lack of interest in favorite activities. It may be more challenging to recognize depression in children with ASDs and other developmental disabilities. When considering depression, it may help to compare your child's current state to how she "typically" acts, paying particular attention to crying spells, enjoyment of activities, interest in being around others, sleep patterns, appetite, and energy level. In children with ASDs and depression, the intensity, frequency, and duration of behaviors such as aggression and irritability may increase from typical levels. Often, there is a family history of depression.

I Have Concerns; What Should I Do?

The best thing you can do if you think your child might have an ASD is to bring up your concerns with your child's pediatrician. By listening to your concerns and observing your child, your pediatrician can work with you to decide on the next step. If your pediatrician shares your concerns and recommends a more complete ASD evaluation, the process will help you learn more about how you can help your child reach his full potential. While getting an ASD diagnosis may be difficult for you and your family, receiving the diagnosis at a young age means you can start early with intervention therapies that will, in the long run, be the best for your child.

Carly, for instance, knew for months that something wasn't right with her son Asher. She was devastated to get the diagnosis but immediately had help from an early intervention therapist who had been in the room when Asher was diagnosed. Carly took a couple of weeks to let the diagnosis sink in and to start figuring out what she needed to do. In the meantime, the therapist registered Asher for early intervention services, which Asher attended a few times before starting at a school for children with special needs 2 months later.

During every one of your child's health supervision visits, your pediatrician may ask about any concerns you may have about your child's behavior or development. Be sure to take these opportunities to talk about any concerns that you or other caregivers may have. Also, inform your pediatrician about any other family members who have ASDs or symptoms of ASDs. Your pediatrician will carefully observe your child and perform an examination. The frequent visits you have with your child's pediatrician will allow for a complete view of your child's overall development.

At your child's 9-, 18-, and 24- or 30-month visits, your pediatrician may ask you to fill out a screening questionnaire about your child's development. Some of these questionnaires will ask about all aspects of your child's development. Others may ask about signs of ASDs. It's important to know that these tools assist your pediatrician in identifying children at risk for developmental disabilities but are not used to diagnose any specific condition. If your child is found to be at risk, he will be referred for a comprehensive evaluation. It is during this evaluation that a specific developmental disorder may be diagnosed.

A comprehensive evaluation for ASDs may involve assessments by several professionals who ideally work as a team. Team members might include your child's pediatrician, a developmental pediatrician, a psychologist, a psychiatrist, a neurologist, a speech-language

---

WORDS TO KNOW

Developmental surveillance: the process your pediatrician uses to identify children who may be at risk for developmental disorders such as autism spectrum disorder (ASD). This involves listening to your concerns about your child's development and behavior, making careful observations of your child during visits, and asking about other family members with developmental disabilities.

Developmental screening: a process your pediatrician uses that involves parental questionnaires (standardized tools) about your child's behavior and development to further clarify if a child is at risk for a developmental disability.

Comprehensive evaluation: A multistep assessment of children who, through surveillance and screening, are found to be at risk for an ASD. It involves questioning caregivers, observing the child, performing a physical examination, and administering any tests that may assist in arriving at a specific diagnosis. Ideally, this is done by a team of professionals.

JACOB'S STORY

A case study in the October 2010 issue of the *Journal of Developmental and Behavioral Pediatrics* recounts the story of Jacob, a 22-month-old boy with no family history of autism. But his parents' answers to 3 questions on a screening test raised concerns. They revealed to their pediatrician that Jacob did not pretend play, such as talking on the phone or taking care of a doll; did not respond to his name when they called; and sometimes stared at nothing or wandered for no purpose. On a different screening test of general development, the parents expressed concerns about Jacob's limited speech. At almost 2 years of age, Jacob spoke only 2 words in Hebrew and 1 in English. Given the results on these 2 screening instruments, Jacob was referred for a diagnostic evaluation to look for developmental problems, autism being just one of them.

---

pathologist, an occupational therapist, a social worker, an audiologist, and others. Each of these professionals has a unique role in the evaluation of a child with a suspected ASD (Table 3-1).

Regardless of exactly who is involved, your child's evaluation should include a health history, a physical examination, careful observation, and a hearing test. In addition, other team members might do more formal evaluations of your child's language and cognition as well as administer other ASD-specific tests. Still other tests may be recommended if it seems that your child's autism is associated with a medical condition such as those listed in Chapter 2. (Table 3-2 on page 63 lists screening tools that pediatricians may use to help refer children for ASDs.)

Even with so many experts and diagnostic tools available, accurately diagnosing a child with an ASD remains a challenge. Because there is not yet a clear biological marker that can be detected in the blood or seen on digital imaging to identify children with ASDs, a lot of factors may complicate an accurate diagnosis. Some of the criteria used to diagnose ASDs are not easily applied to very young children, especially those younger than 2 years. Also, it is not uncommon for families to receive different diagnoses from different evaluators. In addition, it is difficult in some parts of the country to have access to a team of health care professionals with the skills and expertise to diagnose ASDs.

TABLE 3-1. INTERDISCIPLINARY ASSESSMENT TEAM FOR CHILDREN WITH AUTISM SPECTRUM DISORDERS	
Team Member	**Role**
Audiologist	Evaluates for hearing loss as etiology for developmental delay
Developmental pediatrician, child neurologist, physician	Performs medical evaluation Identifies and treats associated conditions
Geneticist and genetic counselor	Performs evaluation when an underlying medical condition or genetic syndrome is suggested by family history, examination, or clinical course Counsels family on recurrence risk
Psychiatrist	Evaluates and treats associated psychiatric conditions and maladaptive behaviors
Psychologist	Administers cognitive or developmental testing Administers diagnostic tools Identifies associated psychiatric conditions and develops behavioral treatment plan
Occupational therapist	Evaluates for fine and gross motor deficits Evaluates for sensory processing deficits Develops plan for treatment
Social worker	Identifies family needs Refers family to formal and informal support agencies and organizations
Speech-language pathologist	Evaluates for expressive, receptive, and pragmatic language deficits Develops plan for treatment

Note: To facilitate recollection of developmental milestones and behavior, parents should review baby books, records, and video recordings of their child's early years before attending a diagnostic evaluation.

Source: Carbone PS, Farley M, Davis T. Primary care for children with autism. *Am Fam Physician.* 2010;81(4):453–460.

TABLE 3-2. SELECTED AUTISM SPECTRUM DISORDER SCREENING QUESTIONNAIRES BY AGE	
Screening Tool	**Ages**
Communication and Symbolic Behavior Scales Developmental Profile Infant-Toddler Checklist (CSBS-DP-ITC)	6–24 months
Modified Checklist for Autism in Toddlers (M-CHAT)	16–48 months
Social Communication Questionnaire (SCQ)	For child 4 years or older (who has developmental skills greater than or equal to 2-year-old)
Childhood Asperger Syndrome Test (CAST)	4–11 years old
Krug Asperger's Disorder Index (KADI)	6–21 years old
Autism Spectrum Screening Questionnaire (ASSQ)	7–16 years old
Autism Spectrum Quotient (AQ)—Adolescent Version	11–16 years old

When the Diagnosis Is Autism Spectrum Disorder

It can be difficult to learn that your child has a lifelong developmental disability. Naturally, you as a parent, other caregivers, and extended family need to grieve about this. You will undoubtedly worry about what the future holds. Keep in mind during these difficult times that most children with ASDs will make significant progress in overall function. Some children with ASDs can do exceptionally well and may even remain in a regular education classroom. Many will have meaningful relationships with family and peers and achieve a good level of independence as adults.

It is important to remember that while an ASD diagnosis may change what you thought your parenting experience would be, we now know that children with ASDs and other developmental disabilities can achieve so much more in life as long as they are given appropriate support and opportunities. Even parents like Carly, who was initially devastated to learn her son had autism, realize now that getting a diagnosis will help them better understand their children and allow them to move forward with finding the right services for them. In the coming chapters we will describe how you can help your child access the support and opportunities that will allow her to reach her full potential.

> **Until recently, our 20-month-old son was always chatty and seemed to be on his way to saying some words. But my husband and I have noticed lately that he isn't speaking as much or doing as much pointing or gesturing as he did just weeks ago. We recently moved to a new house and my husband started a new job with different hours, so he sees less of our son. Could the changes in environment be affecting our son's communication skills? We're worried.**

It's tempting to blame the slowdown in your son's language skills on the move or not seeing as much of his father. But if your child is experiencing noticeable changes in his ability to communicate, you need to bring this to your pediatrician's attention. Your son is at an age when setbacks in language skills may be a sign of autism. Approximately 25% to 30% of children with ASDs appear to be developing normally and then lose some or all of their language and social skills. Discuss your concerns with your child's pediatrician. Getting prompt attention, even without a definitive diagnosis, will allow you to learn how to help your son and gain access to early intervention, which will help him reach his full potential.

Autism Champion: Catherine Lord, PhD

Catherine Lord, PhD, was an undergraduate when she took a psychology class at the University of California, Los Angeles, with Dr O. Ivar Lovaas, the psychologist who helped develop the applied behavior analysis therapy for ASDs. "It was just at the time when he was taking on the challenge of autism as a way to test a theory that operant conditioning could teach anyone anything," Dr Lord recalls.

Dr Lord participated in a project involving teaching children with ASDs to speak. "I worked with 2 children who were so different from each other who also had amazing similarities," she says. "I think that is what captivated me originally. I was also fascinated by the links that people with autism make between ideas and the things they see, even when they cannot easily communicate about them."

Today, Dr Lord is the director of the Center for Autism and the Developing Brain at New York-Presbyterian Hospital, Weill Cornell Medical College, and Columbia University Medical Center. She is credited with devising the Autism Diagnostic Observation Schedule (ADOS), a standardized assessment of communication, social interaction, and play for diagnosing individuals with ASDs. She is also a coauthor of the Autism Diagnostic Interview, which was recently revised (ADI-R), for clinicians to use in interviews with caregivers about a child's early development, communication, social interaction, and patterns of behavior.

The goal, she says, was to create a way to compare children from one center to the next. "We realized that the process by which clinicians made diagnoses was quite different at each center," Dr Lord says. "Even the criteria for diagnosis were different. We wanted to have information about various symptoms of autism so that we could describe participants in a way that anyone could interpret."

The ADI-R and ADOS have been important in providing standardized methods for research on the genetics and neurobiology of ASD. Both instruments have allowed clinicians all over the world to have valid and reliable tools for identifying and specifying the behaviors that we now know as ASDs.

CHAPTER 4

Behavioral and Developmental Treatment

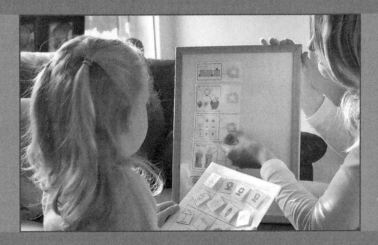

You've just learned that your child has an autism spectrum disorder (ASD). The next step is to find the right treatments or supports for your child, a process that can be challenging and rewarding. The list of potential therapies is complex.

A solid intervention plan is essential to a child with an ASD and can make a significant difference in how well he reaches his full potential. In this chapter, we will take a look at the main developmental and behavioral approaches for treating ASDs, including the earliest forms of intervention that a young child can receive. We will also examine therapies that target specific skills. Keep in mind that there is no single prescription for all children, and at first you may feel overwhelmed by all the options available to you. You'll also get a lot of advice from various experts, family members, and other families of children with ASDs. In the end, choosing the right mix of therapies for your child will take careful thought and consideration. It will also depend on resources in your community and what best suits your entire family, which we'll discuss in later chapters. For now, it's important to know exactly what your options are.

Goals and Management Plan

The main goal of any ASD treatment is to help your child learn the skills he'll need to function in this world. For a child with an ASD, that means helping him gain essential communication and social skills, and eliminating behaviors that are disruptive or unhelpful. It's also important to teach your child how to apply those skills in different situations in ways that are socially appropriate, a process known as *generalization*. In other words, these interventions will help him get along with other children, learn the most he can at school, and master basic daily life skills.

The process won't be easy, and it may take months, even years, for you to see progress, depending on the degree of your child's ASD. But the end goal is this: you want to maximize your child's independence and quality of life and at the same time, alleviate stress on your family. To accomplish this, it will be helpful to meet with your child's pediatrician to assemble a team of professionals who work together to develop and implement a management plan that addresses the needs of your child and family.

What Makes a Good Plan?

Every plan is different, just as every child is unique. And how a child responds to a particular intervention will vary too. Each plan has its own philosophy, practice, and approach. Some are behavioral and focus on teaching your child proper behaviors while minimizing inappropriate ones. Others are relational and use relationship-building skills to improve a child's functioning. Others are educational and emphasize the importance of teaching skills that help a child learn better in school. Still others focus on specific skills such as speech, self-care, and socializing. Others may merge different approaches. You may find it helpful to do more than one program and to change treatments as the needs of your child change. You can observe programs by looking them up on Web sites like www.youtube.com and direct any follow-up questions to your child's pediatrician or a designated expert recommended by her.

Experts from the National Research Council (NRC) agree that some principles and elements are essential to making a young child's intervention program successful. For starters, placing the child into an intervention program is best done as soon as you and your pediatrician suspect he has an ASD, rather than waiting for a definitive diagnosis. Children who receive therapy early generally do better than those who wait. It's important too that the child's management plan is intensive, defined by the NRC as year-round and at least 25 hours a week. It should be carefully planned and deliver developmentally appropriate educational activities that address specific goals. An ideal educational program should have a low student-to-teacher ratio (2:1 or less) so that each child gets plenty of one-on-one time or small-group instruction.

A good plan should also involve other people besides the therapist to reinforce new skills in the routine settings of your child's daily life (known as generalizing new skills). Parents, for instance, should always be part of the process and may even undergo rigorous training to learn how to help their child. Siblings often become part of the process as well as

---

A PRACTICAL POINT

Intervention programs are beneficial for all children. So even if your child is not diagnosed with an autism spectrum disorder, these practices are just as valuable to "typical" children.

grandparents, babysitters, and others involved in the child's care. With school-aged children, teachers may be involved too. In addition, to the extent possible, your child should have opportunities to interact with peers with typical development. (For more information, see Chapter 9.)

An intervention program should provide a great deal of structure. It should have a predictable routine, a visual schedule of activities, and well-defined physical boundaries that minimize distractions. The child should have the opportunity to apply the skills he learns in the program to new environments and situations and have the chance to practice functional skills for daily living. At the same time, it's important that whoever is doing the therapy is measuring and documenting your child's progress. Only by knowing how well your child is doing will you be able to gauge a therapy's effectiveness.

Because ASDs are complex conditions that affect several developmental areas, it's important to put together a management plan that addresses multiple areas of concern, including social skills and communication. In addition to teaching skills you want your child to acquire, it's important to help him eliminate behaviors that are not helpful. Ultimately, you are preparing your child for greater independence and responsibility, be it in the home, at school, or in the community.

It's important to understand that not all children require the same amount of treatment. Just as the condition varies among children, so too does the therapy. High-functioning children, for instance, may need minimal intervention. Children with ASDs who have more prominent symptoms and challenges that interfere with their daily functioning may require several types of treatment at a higher intensity (ie, number of times per week). Some children will need therapies for only a few years, while others may benefit from more prolonged treatment. The majority of children continue to need assistance with independent living, jobs, social relationships, and mental health well into adulthood. Familiarizing yourself with the various options available is key to finding therapies that will work for your child. Your pediatrician can help you become familiar with the different professionals that offer services as part of your child's overall management plan.

The Behavioral Approach: Applied Behavior Analysis

Some of the more well-known ASD therapies use a method known as *applied behavior analysis* (ABA). The principles of ABA are based on the work of B.F. Skinner, a behavioral psychologist in the 1930s who said behavior was manipulated and controlled by events in the physical world. These principles were refined and later used in the 1960s by psychologists and researchers to teach children with autism. It has also been used to teach and modify behaviors in children and adults with other behavioral and developmental challenges. Applied behavior analysis has the most evidence-based support in the scientific literature and is currently regarded as one of the most effective interventions for children with ASDs.

In short, ABA is a method of teaching that uses reinforcement to motivate and shape desired behavior. It begins with a basic understanding of ABC—*antecedent*, *behavior*, and *consequence*.

- *Antecedent* is the verbal or physical drive, such as a direct request from mom, that precedes the behavior.
- *Behavior* is the child's response to the antecedent. If mom asks him to point to an apple and he does, he is demonstrating an appropriate behavioral response to the antecedent.
- *Consequence* is what happens after the child performs the behavior. The type of consequence determines whether the behavior will occur again in the future or gradually diminish. Positive reinforcement—praise and a mother's smile, for example—is more likely to ensure that the child will point to the apple the next time mom asks.

Traditional ABA, sometimes called the Lovaas Model, grew out of research in the early 1970s by O. Ivar Lovaas, PhD. By the mid-1980s, Dr Lovaas was able to demonstrate in his research that using ABA in intensive and early interventions for ASDs enabled almost half of the children to succeed in regular education classrooms. Even children who do not move on to regular classrooms can still benefit from ABA, just as parents can use ABA methods to teach and manage their child's behavior. Studies have shown that children who receive intensive ABA therapies may be able to make significant and sustained gains in IQ, language, academic performance, and self-care behaviors. They also can make notable strides in social skills.

The goal of ABA is simple: increase the behaviors that you want your child to do and decrease those that are undesirable and troublesome. To achieve this, it's important that your child work with a skilled therapist who will break down the skills and behaviors into small, measurable steps. Desired behavior is then taught using repeated trials, with desired behaviors reinforced with positive rewards that your child finds highly motivating. Your child should also have the opportunity to practice these behaviors in a variety of settings, such as the home, school, and the community.

Applied behavior analysis has been used in many settings for different purposes and can be used for people with ASDs to teach communication, play, self-care, work, social, academic, and community living skills. The original therapy by Dr Lovaas delivered 40 hours a week of one-on-one work with a trained professional. However, many experts now believe that less intensive interventions can work just as well. Your child's treatment team will recommend the most appropriate intensity based on your child's needs.

To determine exactly what your child needs, your therapist may recommend doing a *functional behavioral analysis* (FBA). An FBA identifies antecedents and consequences surrounding a specific behavior, one you want to encourage or one that you'd like to eliminate. The FBA can suggest strategies for intervening that will alter the behavior and ways to gauge whether the intervention is working. Although you may hear more about this assessment tool in the context of a school setting—especially when there are problematic behaviors— an FBA can also be used as part of ABA.

Discrete Trial Teaching

One of the most widely used ABA therapies is known as discrete trial teaching (DTT). Discrete trial teaching is often used to teach basic skills such as paying attention, following directions, and imitating instructions. A trained instructor works one-on-one with a child, who is given an instruction or request, which is technically known as a *discriminative stimulus*. If the child performs the request, the instructor praises him for what he did and may even give him a reward that he finds immensely enjoyable.

Here's how DTT works: Let's say you want to teach your child to say hello when he sees other people. The instructor would explain and demonstrate to the child that he needs to say hello when the instructor enters the room. Walking into the room is the antecedent, and your child saying hello is the behavior. Each time your child says hello, he is praised by the instructor and given a reward, such as a sticker, which is the consequence. If your child does not say hello, the therapist may help your child by having him repeat a hello that the therapist says. This extra help in demonstrating correct behavior is called a prompt. The scenario is then repeated until your child masters this skill. Learning is successful when the child follows the request independently, without any prompts. To make sure your child has absorbed the lesson, the sequence of instructions may be done many times in different settings to make sure the behavior has been generalized.

Keep in mind that the instruction may be delivered verbally, in a visual such as a picture, or with a gesture such as pointing. However it's given, it should be done so clearly, concisely, and in a way that is easily understood by your child.

Formal DTT is often done in sessions that last 2 or 3 hours, with sessions for young children being done at a small desk with a therapist. Each session consists of short periods of structured time devoted to a single task with short breaks throughout the session.

Critics of DTT say the method does not teach children spontaneity and that the behaviors learned in such a highly structured setting aren't easily transferred to a child's natural environment. To address these concerns, there are other methods using ABA that are considered more natural.

Incidental Teaching

Shaping a child's behavior can sometimes involve placing her in a situation that forces her to do something. For instance, you might seat a child at a table with paper and no crayons, which would compel her to ask you for the crayons. If you hold a child's favorite toy without offering it to her, you will force her to ask you to give it to her. The lessons the child acquires are taught incidentally, without instruction.

Pivotal Response Treatment

Instead of targeting a specific skill, pivotal response treatment (PRT) (previously called natural language paradigm) focuses on developing overarching, or pivotal, behaviors that affect other behaviors such as motivation, initiating communication with others, and self-management. By improving these broad behaviors, PRT indirectly improves play skills, social behaviors, and the ability to control one's own behavior.

Unlike DTT, which uses a more specific curriculum, PRT is child-directed and taps into the child's natural instinct and desire to interact with adults. It uses rewards and reinforcements tailored specifically to the individual child and involves parents on a regular basis in the child's most natural setting: her home.

Verbal Behavior

Using the same principles of ABA, verbal behavior (VB) works by encouraging the child to use language to get what he wants. Treatment is based on a book by the same title written by B.F. Skinner in 1957. The treatment breaks down language into 4 units—Skinner called them *operants*—each with its own function and purpose. Children who have ASDs often use words as labels, or *tacts*. When a word is used to request something, it is called a *mand*. If the word is being used in a discussion when the object is not there, it's said to be *intra-verbal language*. When a word is repeated, it is called an *echoic*.

The goals of VB are to teach different ways to use language and encourage the child to make greater use of language to make requests and have discussions. The theory behind VB is that knowing language is different from using language.

Treatments Focusing on Relationships

Not everyone believes that focusing on changing behaviors (as in ABA) is the key to treating ASDs. Some well-respected experts believe in relationship-focused methods for treatment. Because social dysfunction is a core feature of ASDs, these experts believe that improving a child's relationships with his caregivers, including parents, teachers, and therapists, is key to overcoming many challenges of ASDs. Among the most common treatments are the Developmental, Individual Difference, Relationship-based (DIR)/Floortime Model and Relationship Development Intervention (RDI).

DIR/Floortime

DIR/Floortime works on the principle that a child's emotional development is the basis of her capacity for learning. Healthy emotional development leads to the ability to engage with others, communicate with purpose, and play in a meaningful way. Floortime is the most common technique used in the DIR model of treatment.

The DIR Model describes an intervention and philosophy created by Stanley Greenspan, MD, and Serena Wieder, PhD. Drs Greenspan and Wieder said children must achieve 6 developmental milestones, which form the foundation for all learning and development, for proper emotional and intellectual growth. These milestones are the abilities to

- Regulate their response to the sensory world and stay calm.
- Engage and relate to others in an intimate and loving way.
- Participate in 2-way communication.
- Communicate in more complex ways, using gestures first and later words to express desires.
- Create emotional ideas.
- Develop emotional and logical thinking.

In children who do not have ASDs, these milestones unfold naturally. But children with ASDs often need treatment to help spur these processes along. Floortime is a therapeutic technique that does exactly what the name implies: it brings the therapist or parent down to the floor to meet the child at her level. Therapy follows a child's natural interests, affect, and emotions. Treatment is individually tailored to the child's developmental level—socially, emotionally, and intellectually—and takes into account how the child experiences the sensory world. The idea is to play with the child by following her lead and at the same time engage her in a way that is warm and inviting.

Like ABA, the goal in DIR/Floortime is to help your child learn to regulate her own behavior, engage with other people, and communicate effectively. Floortime sessions typically last 20 to 30 minutes at a time and may be combined with and applied to other forms of therapy. Over time, activities become more complex.

Relationship Development Intervention

Relationship Development Intervention is a relatively new treatment created by Steven Gutstein, PhD, and Rachelle Sheely, PhD. It focuses on activities that encourage social interaction and motivate the child to become more interested in interpersonal exchanges. According to Dr Gutstein, people who have ASDs tend to withdraw because they are overwhelmed with sensory information. As a result, they prefer what is called *static systems,* such as memorizing facts and rigid rituals and routines, to dynamic systems such as social relationships and complex thinking, which are characterized by unpredictability.

The RDI program targets what the doctors describe as the 6 main deficits of ASDs.

- *Emotional referencing:* The ability to learn from the experiences of others.
- *Social coordination:* The ability to observe and continually regulate one's behavior to engage in meaningful relationships with others.
- *Declarative language:* The ability to use verbal and nonverbal language to interact with other people.
- *Flexible thinking:* The ability to quickly adapt strategies in the face of changing circumstances.
- *Relational information processing:* The ability to obtain meaning from information in the context of something larger. This skill includes solving problems with no right-and-wrong solutions.
- *Foresight and hindsight:* The ability to reflect on the past and anticipate potential future scenarios in a way that is productive and helpful.

Relationship Development Intervention is administered primarily by parents but also by teachers and other professionals. Parents learn the program through training seminars, books, and other materials and work with an RDI-certified consultant. It begins with family-guided participation, in which the child works one-on-one with the parent. Everyday tasks like preparing rice, watering flowers, and cleaning a sink can be used in RDI. The program relies less on verbal instructions and more on visuals, including facial expressions, to encourage eye contact and nonverbal communication to engage the child in joint tasks.

In the second phase, known as the dynamic education program, lessons become more challenging and complex. The curriculum combines developing mental processes with traditional academic training and real-world problem solving. As children progress through the program, they are encouraged to use these skills in settings that are increasingly unfamiliar and distracting. The child may learn from making mistakes as well as how to evaluate contradicting information and handle misunderstandings.

So far, the effectiveness of RDI has not been conclusively proven scientifically but is mainly based on personal experiences.

Social Communication, Emotional Regulation, and Transactional Support Model

The Social Communication, Emotional Regulation, and Transactional Support (SCERTS) Model borrows from several of the previously described approaches. It also uses methods from the Treatment and Education of Autistic and Related Communication-Handicapped Children (TEACCH) program (see Chapter 5). Not surprisingly, SCERTS is the brainchild of a multidisciplinary team of experts: Barry Prizant, PhD; Amy Wetherby, PhD; Emily Rubin, MS; and Amy C. Laurent.

The name refers to the following 3 primary areas of focus:

- *Social communication* refers to spontaneous, functional communication; emotional expression; and secure and trusting relationships with other people. The goal is to help the child become more confident and even to enjoy the social interactions she has with adults and other children. To do that, the model emphasizes joint attention abilities and symbolic behavior. *Joint attention* is the ability to share attention, emotions, and intentions in a give-and-take fashion. At a more sophisticated level, it's the ability to share experiences, stay on topic, and consider a listener's level of interest. *Symbolic behavior* refers to communicating with others through means beyond just speech, so the child may have other strategies for making her desires and intentions known, such as gestures or visuals. The belief is that when kids have greater mastery of these skills, they will come to enjoy the company of other people.

- *Emotional regulation* is the ability to regulate one's emotional state, even in the face of everyday stressors. It is the ability to be fully present for learning, interacting with others, and participating in activities. Children with ASDs are often "too high" or "too low" in their arousal, which can make it hard for them to focus. Unexpected changes in circumstances, for instance, can provoke intense anxiety in children with ASDs who prefer routines and rituals and make it hard for them to remain calm. The goal of the emotional regulation aspect of SCERTS is to help the child adapt and cope with life's daily challenges that upset her state of arousal.

- *Transactional support* is the development and implementation of supports that help partners—parents, teachers, or siblings—respond to the child's needs at a given moment. It's about the things that other people can do to modify and adapt a child's environment so that she is better able to learn and perform everyday activities. It might involve interpersonal support from peers who help create positive friendships, or it might include a teacher's visual aids in a classroom to help with learning.

In the SCERTS Model, all parties come together to make sure the child has the optimal situation for relating to peers, learning, and engaging in activities. Unlike more regimented ABA treatments or child-driven approaches of DIR/Floortime, SCERTS strives to be systematic and semi-structured but flexible. Activities are designed to be consistent and predictable but also meaningful to the individual child, who gets to share control of activities. While the parent or teacher can make the most of teachable moments, the child can also assert her motivation.

The SCERTS Model is usually done in a school setting by SCERTS-trained special education teachers or speech therapists. The underlying belief is that children learn best with and from other children, who serve as models of good communication and social behavior. Family members are typically given information or direct instructions on how to help a child progress in developing her skills. To determine whether a child is benefiting from the program, teachers or therapists can use the SCERTS assessment process, which involves observations and reports from caregivers.

When Autism Spectrum Disorder Is Suspected Early

It was once believed that children who have ASDs couldn't be diagnosed until they were toddlers or beyond. In recent years, it's become apparent that signs of ASDs usually appear in the first 2 years of a child's life. In 2007, the American Academy of Pediatrics began recommending universal screening of all children at their 18- and 24-month well-child visits. Looking for signs of ASDs at this young age meant that it was important for parents to have options for therapy and to have this therapy start as soon as possible.

Early Intervention

If the screening shows that a child is at risk for a developmental disorder, he should be referred to the state early intervention (EI) program. The EI Program is a federal grant program run by individual states under Part C of the Individuals with Disabilities Education Act that works with children from birth until their third birthday. It is also called the Program for Infants and Toddlers with Disabilities. Although the program exists in all 50 states, eligibility for the program and types of services varies by state. The program targets children who show a delay in cognitive, social, or communication skills. They may also have a delay in physical or motor abilities or self-care skills. Anyone can refer a child to EI, including a pediatrician, parents, grandparents, or a child care provider. The child doesn't even need a diagnosis. The EI program's team of specialists will test and evaluate the child to see if he qualifies for the program.

If, after the initial evaluation, your child is eligible for the program, you will receive an Individualized Family Service Program (IFSP), which explains the services recommended for your child and how EI will help you and your family support your child. The IFSP will describe your child's current developmental levels, ways to improve your child's development, and the outcomes you can expect. It will also outline the specific services that you and your family will receive and the goal dates for starting and ending those services. In addition, the IFSP will provide information on how EI will help the child and family transition to school services when the child turns 3. The IFSP should be developed with the family's values in mind and be supportive of the family's routine and priorities.

Service providers in an EI program include many types of professionals such as social workers, speech therapists, occupational therapists (OTs), physical therapists, registered dietitians, developmental therapists, and psychologists. Services may be provided in your home or in the community.

Like the program itself, payment for EI varies from state to state. Some states provide services at no charge, while others charge according to family income. But all states must provide certain services free of charge, including screening, multidisciplinary evaluations, referrals for service needs, and coordination of services. Development, review, and evaluation of the IFSP is also free of charge.

Experts agree that EI is an essential component in the early treatment of ASDs and other developmental problems. The program has been shown to be beneficial to socially disadvantaged children who don't have an ASD and often leads to less need for special education services for those children later on. Early intervention also helps overall family function and improves outcomes for children who have a biologically based disorder such as an ASD.

Early Start Denver Model: New Evidence for Treating Young Children With Autism Spectrum Disorders

Until recent years, children younger than 2 years who were suspected of having ASDs or diagnosed with ASDs had few options for treatment. That began to change in the 1980s. Among the most compelling and effective methods for treating young children is the Early Start Denver Model (ESDM), which uses play with a teacher or parent to teach a host of developmental skills. These skills cover all areas of early development: cognitive skills, language, social behavior, imitation, fine and gross motor skills, self-help skills, and adaptive behavior. The ESDM was created by Sally J. Rogers, PhD, who had helped to develop the Denver Model for preschoolers while at the University of Colorado. The ESDM draws on the methods of the Denver Model and is based on the principles of ABA. In particular, it uses PRT to teach communication, cognitive, and language skills. The ESDM may be used for children as young as 12 months (and is now being tested on even younger infants with ASD-like features) with the overall goal of promoting the child's social and communication development. Though ESDM encompasses several areas of skill development, it is especially focused on teaching the child imitation, nonverbal communication (including joint attention), verbal communication, social behaviors, and play.

During an ESDM session, a child will be engaged in a joint activity with a therapist or her parent where there is constant give-and-take and turn-taking between the therapist and child. Activities are designed around what interests the child and uses objects found in a child's natural environment. That might mean playing patty-cake with the child or rolling a ball back and forth. The ESDM is considered an intense intervention and may involve up to 20 to 25 hours of intervention a week (which may include time working with the parents and child together). The interaction is intended to be emotionally positive, even fun, and is designed to coax the child to become more social. But instead of keeping a child in a classroom or a therapist's office, these playful lessons can be delivered by therapists and parents alike so that the child is engaged with a responsive caregiver throughout her day.

The ESDM relies heavily on parental involvement and reinforces what child development experts already know: parents play a major role in the development of their children's social, language, and communication skills, whether or not a child has an ASD. In the child with an ASD who is undergoing ESDM, parents become co-therapists. Parents are taught to spot teachable moments throughout the day, help their child practice developing skills at appropriate times, and work with their child to eliminate unwanted behaviors. The ESDM program should be woven seamlessly into the child's day during mealtimes, family outings, dressing, bathing, toileting, and bedtime. Ideally, parents should devote at least an hour or two each day to working with their child while she is undergoing ESDM. Eventually, siblings may be brought in to participate as a way to help the child develop social skills with peers.

Research has found the ESDM to be highly effective. A 2009 study showed that using ESDM resulted in significant improvements in young children diagnosed with ASDs. The study looked at 48 children between 18 and 30 months of age who were diagnosed with an ASD. The children were randomly assigned to 1 of 2 groups: one received ESDM for 2 years, and the other was referred to community providers for services. After 2 years, the children who received ESDM had greater improvements in IQ, communication skills, and language abilities than the kids who were referred to community services. The children receiving ESDM also had better daily living skills, motor skills, and adaptive behaviors. In addition, the children who underwent ESDM were more likely to have a change in their diagnosis from ASD to pervasive developmental disorder–not otherwise specified.

Specific Therapies to Develop Skills

Treatments described in this chapter are geared specifically to children who have ASDs, but these children often require other treatments to address problems with speech, self-care skills, and sensory processing issues. Children may also benefit from group and individual social skills training.

Speech-Language Therapy

Because social communication difficulty is a core feature of ASD, most children with ASDs will benefit from some form of speech-language therapy to communicate more effectively in social situations. As stated earlier, some children with ASDs will have great difficulty communicating their wants and needs, while others may talk nearly constantly with advanced speech like "little professors." Teaching children with ASDs to communicate with others in social situations involves comprehension and expression. The extent of therapy varies widely from one child to the next, but many children with ASDs can benefit from speech-language therapy.

The exact services your child requires is determined after evaluation by a speech-language pathologist, often called a speech therapist. Therapy itself may be done individually, in a small-group setting, or in a classroom. However, therapy is most effective when it involves everyone—teachers, support staff, families, and even the child's peers—to encourage the child to use speech and language skills in a natural setting throughout the day.

It's important to think of language as being more than speech. Because some children with ASDs become frustrated about not being able to verbally communicate their wants and needs, they may benefit from augmentative communication—using gestures, sign language, and picture communication programs. In particular, your child may benefit from the Picture Exchange Communication System, a method that uses ABA principles to teach children with less developed verbal abilities to communicate with pictures. With guidance from a therapist, teacher, or parent, the child learns how to exchange a picture for an object and eventually learns to use pictures to express thoughts and desires. Eventually, the child learns to create sentences using more than one picture and to answer questions.

Introducing augmentative communication to nonverbal children with ASDs does not keep them from learning to talk, and there is some evidence that they may be more stimulated to learn speech if they already understand something about symbolic communication. Augmentative communication may also include the use of electronic devices, some of which have synthesized speech output.

Social Skills

Difficulty interacting with other people is a key challenge for children with ASDs, and teaching social skills can be a critical part of any intervention. Of particular benefit is joint attention training, which may be especially important in children who are not yet speaking. Joint attention, the sharing of experiences, comes before the development of later social language abilities and can predict how well a child develops those skills. In fact, studies show that functional speech and language typically starts about a year after a child masters joint attention.

Symbolic play skills, or pretend play, are another important component of social skills. A 2006 study found that children who were in a joint attention or symbolic play intervention group had better social play interactions afterward than children who did not receive these interventions.

A good social skills intervention teaches children how to respond to friendly overtures from other children and adults, initiate social interactions, and minimize stereotypic behavior. It also teaches them how to use and manage a broad variety of social skills. A typical training session may teach children something as basic as how to make eye contact or something more challenging like how to invite a friend over to play. Social skills training can take many different forms. Lessons are usually taught by social workers, speech therapists, or psychologists, using a variety of methods such as storytelling, visual cueing, games, video modeling, and role-playing.

Formal social skills curricula do exist, but many of these activities can be done informally in the home with the family. In fact, the family plays a critical role in daily interactions that can teach joint attention and social communication. These interactions can be easily woven into the child's daily activities and should begin even before a diagnosis is made. It's also important for the child to have a wealth of opportunities to engage with peers with typical development. For information on how parents can encourage social skills, see Chapter 12.

Occupational Therapy

Children with ASDs often have deficits in the areas of fine motor skills, sensory processing, and motor planning. These can show up as difficulties with basic self-care skills such as getting dressed, using a spoon, or brushing teeth. Some have trouble with play skills, such as building puzzles or using scissors, and basic life skills, such as sitting still in a classroom. Occupational therapists often can help with these issues. An OT evaluates the child's fine motor skills and sensory processing development and prepares strategies for learning tasks of daily living. These interventions may be delivered in sessions with a therapist and then practiced at home and school. Goals will depend on the needs of the individual child, but occupational therapy strives to help children gain more independence and live a higher quality of life.

Sensory Integration Therapy

Sensory integration is a term that has been used to describe processes in the brain that allow us to take information we receive from our 5 senses, organize it, and respond appropriately. We also have a vestibular sense (balance) that tells us how to position our bodies and heads, and a proprioceptive sense (awareness of body in space) that helps us know what we do with our joints, muscles, and ligaments. In children who have ASDs, sensory processing deficits have been theorized to cause difficulties that affect behavior and life skills. As a result, some children may be hypersensitive or hyposensitive to stimuli in the surroundings. Loud music, for instance, may cause intense discomfort, while bright fluorescent lights that bother others may be riveting to some children with ASDs. Children with sensory processing deficits may have difficulty with motor skills, balance, and eye-hand coordination. Some children will look for ways to seek out certain sensations and engage in self-stimulating behaviors like rocking back and forth, head banging, and oral exploration of nonedible objects.

Sensory integration therapy, which was developed in the 1970s by an OT, A. Jean Ayres, is designed to help children with sensory-processing problems (including possibly those with ASDs) cope with the difficulties they have processing sensory input. Therapy sessions are play-oriented and may include using equipment such as swings, trampolines, and slides.

Sensory integration also uses therapies such as deep pressure, brushing, weighted vests, and swinging. These therapies appear to sometimes be able to calm an anxious child. In addition, sensory integration therapy is believed to increase a child's threshold for tolerating sensory-rich environments, make transitions less disturbing, and reinforce positive behaviors.

Although there are scientific studies to show that children with ASDs are more likely to have sensory-processing problems, the effectiveness of sensory integration therapy as a therapy for ASDs is limited and inconclusive. While this does not mean that the therapy might not be helpful in some children, effectiveness so far is mainly based on personal experiences. Talk with your child's pediatrician if you suspect that your child has difficulties with sensory processing; there may be resources in the community for further evaluation.

You may also learn about auditory integration training or behavioral optometry as methods for controlling sensory input. Both treatments aim to alter the child's response to sensory stimuli, but neither method has proved to be scientifically valid. Also, there is no evidence that any problems seen with ASDs are related to these auditory or visual problems. (See Chapter 7.)

What's Next?

Now that you have at least some understanding of the many treatments for ASDs, you may be wondering where to go for help. The answer varies, depending on the age of your child and services available in your community. A good place to start is with your child's pediatrician. You can also find information through local chapters of national organizations such as those listed in Appendix A. Another good resource is other parents who have already begun this journey.

In general, if your child is younger than 3 years, you can access many of these services through the EI program. Children aged 3 to 21 years access services through the special education department of the local school district, starting with the special services coordinator at your home school. Your school district will be a vital resource of information, as you will see in the next chapter.

Autism Champion: Kirsten Sneid

When Kirsten Sneid learned her son Evan had severe autism, she was devastated. But she was determined to find a way to connect with him. "I never asked why, why him, or why us," she says. "If I went down that road, I don't think I'd ever get out of there. Instead, I prayed. What now? Where now? Who now?"

She started by abandoning her nursing career to raise Evan and his older brother Ian, who had been diagnosed with pervasive developmental disorder–not otherwise specified. She began hosting wine parties and coffee hours at her home, where she brought together other parents of children with ASDs. In 2001, she became the founding president of the Autism Society in her county to help improve services for children with ASDs. "It started as a support group," she says. "We were constantly knocking on the doors of community service providers. We realized that this was a community health care crisis that required a community response." The group is now called the Autism Society of the Heartland.

Obstacles arose at every turn. When Evan hit preschool, Kirsten realized there were no good preschool programs for kids like him. So she created an ABA program in her home and hired college students who were studying occupational therapy and speech and language pathology. The program was so successful that the local school district used it to create its own. Kirsten also joined the Kansas Coalition for Autism Legislation and lobbied legislators for insurance coverage for ASD services. She helped organize think tanks like the Greater Kansas City Autism Initiative and served on numerous advisory boards, including the Thompson Center for Autism and Neurodevelopmental Disabilities at the University of Missouri and the Kansas Center for Autism Research and Training at the University of Kansas.

These days, Evan is 16 years old with limited verbal skills. At 18, Ian is a student at a local community college and no longer on the spectrum. And Kirsten has returned to her nursing career and is serving on the board of Expanding College for Exceptional Learners, or EXCEL. The group helps provide funding to bistate colleges willing to create educational opportunities for postsecondary students with intellectual disabilities. "It's up to the university to put it together, but we help them succeed," she says.

Kirsten says all she ever wanted was to help families of children with ASDs know they are not alone. "I am really just a worker ant who has had the pleasure and the privilege to surround myself with brilliant, motivated people wanting to create change," she says. "And we have."

CHAPTER 5

Tapping Educational Services

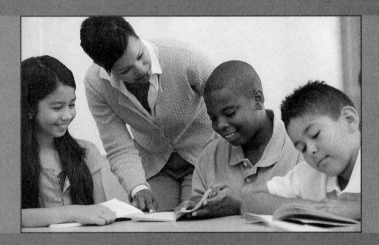

Participating in a traditional school setting can be challenging for children who have an autism spectrum disorder (ASD). Anxiety, fixation on routines, difficulties with sensory input, and the need to perform repetitive behaviors make it a challenge for many children with ASDs to absorb what they're taught or sit still through a lesson. Compounding the difficulties are the social challenges many children with ASDs experience. But with the right accommodations, going to school can be fun, rewarding, and worthwhile for children who have ASDs. In fact, under federal law, all children, including those with disabilities like autism, are entitled to a free and appropriate education. That means your child may be able to receive special education, a program of instruction that is tailored to your child's special needs and places him in a setting that will help him make progress.

Special education services begin once a child turns 3 years old with the move from early intervention (EI) programs into early childhood special education (ECSE) programs (developmental preschools) and then to grade school. Special education continues to be available until an eligible child is 21 years old. You already learned about the many kinds of behavioral and developmental services that your child may receive in Chapter 4. Those same services may also be provided in school, as part of your child's special education services. In most cases, your child will receive a mix of these services.

In this chapter, we'll take a look at what you can expect when your child transitions from EI to ECSE and then to grade school. We'll also help you understand some of the teaching strategies that might work best for children who have ASDs. While the teachers, administrators, and staff at your school will play an important role in how well your child does there, you are an important part of the team as well. As is true with children with typical development, parents play an important role in their child's academic success. That is especially true in the case of children with disabilities like autism, where parental input, guidance, and oversight are essential to a child's progress.

Know Your Rights: A Word About the Individuals With Disabilities Education Act

First enacted in 1975 and most recently revised in 2004 (as of this writing), the Individuals with Disabilities Education Act (IDEA) is a law that ensures that all children with disabilities have access to "free and appropriate education in the least restrictive environment." The act governs how states and public agencies provide EI, special education, and related services to more than 6.5 million eligible infants, toddlers, children, and youth with disabilities, including those with ASDs. Infants and toddlers between the ages of birth and 2 years receive EI services under IDEA Part C. Children and youth between the ages of 3 and 21 years receive special education and related services under IDEA Part B.

Federal law places a great deal of emphasis on parental involvement and stresses the importance of including parents in decisions about their children's education. Before a school district identifies the need for highly specialized and individual instruction as part of a child's education program, it must provide prior written notice to, and obtain consent from, the child's parents. The district must also provide parents with information about their rights under IDEA Part B. In addition, parents must work together with school personnel to determine services that the child will receive to meet her unique needs.

First Things First: The All-Important Individualized Education Program

To determine exactly which services your child needs, you will work with a team of specialists to complete a written document known as the Individualized Education Program (IEP). Every child who receives special education services must have an IEP. The IEP is the educational road map for children with disabilities. It spells out your child's goals and outlines the exact education, services, and supplementary aids that the school district will provide for your child.

Parents who feel their child might benefit from special education services should request an IEP evaluation in writing. Your pediatrician can also help draft a letter of request. Parents should work with personnel from their child's EI program to help with this transition. You can begin this process when your child turns 2.

An IEP is written after an evaluation. During the evaluation, current performance levels are established and documented. To be eligible for special education services, your child must be identified with a recognized disability (there are 14 different disability categories under IDEA) and the disability must adversely affect her educational performance.

Every IEP should have several key pieces of information. It should include your child's current levels of performance, measureable goals for the school year, and when reports about her progress will be provided. It should also discuss how well she's able to function in school, how your child will be included with peers with typical development, and how your child will be assessed on statewide and district-wide tests. In addition, should your child qualify for extended school year services, the IEP should lay out the kinds of interventions that your child should receive when school is not in session. The IEP establishes dates and locations of when services will begin, where they will be held, and how long they will last. The IEP should also discuss what will be done when your child's needs change. In addition, the IEP may outline whether your child gets "related services" such as special transportation, speech therapy, occupational therapy, and counseling.

The IEP is written collaboratively by a group—often called an IEP team—made up of the child's parents, a regular education teacher, a special education teacher, psychologists, therapists, a school administrator, and possibly other school personnel. A meeting to discuss the IEP must be held within 30 days after a school determines that a child needs special education services. Parents may invite anyone to this meeting, including personnel such as an advocate or the child's case manager from the EI program. The IEP is evaluated at least every year to determine whether goals are being met and may be adjusted if your child's needs change.

Unfortunately, research has found that many IEPs for children with ASDs are lacking and do not meet recommendations of the National Research Council or requirements of IDEA. Many IEPs omit important information and may not provide services to a child outside of the traditional school year. Many do not adequately describe how goals are to be measured or how certain goals will help the child in school. Many IEPs also fail to say how teachers intend to motivate the child or how they would engage the child in developmentally appropriate tasks or play. Many IEPs do not include parent concerns.

When formulating your child's IEP with your school district, it's important to know exactly what your rights are and what to do if you are not happy with the resulting IEP. Before going to your first IEP meeting, do your research. Become familiar with your state's education laws, and know the types of interventions available to your child based on her needs. A good book to start with is *Educating Children with Autism,* published by the Committee on Educational Interventions for Children with Autism of the National Research Council. You may also want to visit the US Department of Education one-stop shop for resources related to IDEA and rules and regulations concerning the IEP process at http://idea.ed.gov. See Appendix A for more information.

A PARENT'S STORY: BARBARA

Having 2 boys with autism prompted Barbara to do a lot of research into interventions. She came to the conclusion that for her family, applied behavior analysis (ABA) was the best therapy. But when she learned ABA wasn't a therapy option in her school district, she decided to fight for its inclusion in her son's Individualized Education Program.

"As the parent of a child with autism, you have to learn to negotiate. You have to be persuasive and positive. You have to prepare for a legal fight but hope you don't have to. You have to keep good records.

"I always brought solutions to the table, too. When they asked who should be my son's teaching aide [TA], I told them I had someone in mind. When the room he was using for speech therapy got taken away, I told them I didn't care if they used a closet. In fact, he did wind up in a small room without windows.

"Of course, you also have to realize that you won't always get your way. For instance, I wanted them to assess Sam's ability to work in a group. But the TA wasn't willing to take that data, and I had to be willing to put [up] with that."

The bottom line, according to Barbara, is that schools are required to meet your children's needs. "As the parent of a child with autism, I didn't care if I had to beg and grovel for what was important to me. It was for my sons."

The TEACCH Method

In the 1960s, Eric Schopler and his colleagues at the University of North Carolina created an educational approach for teaching children with ASDs known as Treatment and Education of Autistic and Related Communication-Handicapped Children, or TEACCH. Schopler believed that autism was a lifelong disability but that things could be done to help a child adapt to the school and community. The program uses a variety of strategies to accommodate the needs of children with autism and also includes elements of different behavioral and developmental interventions, including applied behavior analysis; Developmental, Individual Difference, Relationship-based (DIR)/Floortime Model; and social skills training. The program stresses the importance of identifying individual strengths and weaknesses and uses structured teaching methods that play to the child's strengths and interests. In particular for children with ASDs, it focuses on 4 main concepts to enhance learning.

- *The organization of the child's physical environment.* The layout of a classroom—where the furniture is placed, the boundaries between work and play areas, and how items are labeled—is critical to how well a child with an ASD learns. TEACCH stresses the importance of creating an environment that minimizes distractions. Work areas, for instance, should not be placed near windows. Leisure areas should not be located near exits. Pieces of tape may be placed on the floor to show where chairs should be situated while seated. The TEACCH method encourages teachers to create an environment with a lot of visual cues that will help children with ASDs better understand directions and rules, transition from one task to another, and remain focused on the activity at hand.
- *A predictable, though flexible, routine.* Students with ASDs have a strong need for consistency and routine. Many of them experience high levels of anxiety if those routines are disrupted, which can interfere with their learning. Providing a clearly illustrated (visuals are always best) schedule helps a child know what to expect in his day.
- *Structured activity systems.* Children with ASDs thrive on structure and like it when tasks that are expected of them are clearly laid out. It's important to create a step-by-step process that's easy for them to understand. Early on, the system might be a series of pictures showing what tasks need to be done and in what order. Later, the system might involve the use of simple words or phrases. In some cases, the task may be arranged from left to

right. As with any system, however, the student should be closely supervised by an adult, such as an aide, or the teacher.

- *An emphasis on visual learning.* Children with ASDs do much better with visual cues, such as pictures, than they do with verbal or auditory ones. A visual schedule with pictures, for instance, may be helpful for outlining the day's activities. Color-coding subject areas can help a student stay organized. A chart with photographs or cartoons may show a child options for appropriate behavior when a classroom gets too noisy. Colored floor mats help him know where to sit for certain activities.

TEACCH is one of the oldest and most widely used programs in schools, and in North Carolina it has been the official form of publicly funded education for children with ASDs since 1978. Although no other state abides by the principles of TEACCH as closely, elements of the program have seeped into classrooms throughout the world.

National Professional Development Center

In 2007, the National Professional Development Center on Autism Spectrum Disorders (NPDC) was founded with funding by the US Department of Education Office of Special Education Programs. It is a multi-university program, and among its goals is to promote evidence-based practice—meaning effective treatments based on scientific research—for children and adolescents with ASDs. The NPDC works with states to provide professional development to teachers and practitioners who serve individuals from birth through 22 years of age with ASDs.

Using very strict criteria, the NPDC does an extensive literature review to determine which studies would be effective for a given service provider. The NPDC then develops a variety of resources and materials, including online modules and implementation checklists, giving service providers access to evidence-based practices. The NPDC updates the literature review periodically so that it reflects recent research and keeps practices current.

Included in evidence-based practices are structured teaching as well as interventions discussed in Chapter 4. To learn more, visit http://autismpdc.fpg.unc.edu.

Teaching Children With Autism Spectrum Disorders

Educating a child with an ASD is not like teaching children with typical development. As you now know, children with ASDs process information differently. Exactly where and how a child is educated in a school varies widely, depending on the child's needs, age, and what is available in your school district. Some children may require a self-contained special education classroom, while others may be included in a mainstream class with peers who do not have ASDs. Often, children who have ASDs have a mix of specialized and inclusive experiences at school. But even the highest functioning students often still need special supports to help them with organization, assignment comprehension, and other essential skills such as learning to manage social and peer relationships.

Every child's educational experiences will vary, just as the difficulties and talents of a child will differ. But like children with typical development, those who have ASDs will have some general concerns that apply to each grade level.

Preschool

Between the ages of 3 and 5 years, your child will most likely attend a preschool program for young children identified under IDEA Part B (Section 619) and often referred to as ECSE programs. These are typically half-day programs. Depending on your child's level of ability, she may be placed in a self-contained classroom, which is made up only of other children with special needs, with a small student-to-teacher ratio and where services such as speech-language therapy, occupational therapy, and social work are integrated into the classroom experience. If appropriate and available, she may be in a blended classroom where she will be part of a class with children who have disabilities and those who do not. In a blended classroom, she may have a higher ratio of students to teachers, and she will be exposed to peers with typical development. She may also have the opportunity to receive specific therapies, such as speech-language or occupational, but these may be pullout services and not implemented directly within the classroom setting.

For some high-functioning children with ASDs, parents and educators may choose to place them in a mainstream preschool, where they are exposed entirely to typically developing children. Specific therapies may be delivered privately after school in the home or community, or they may be done by an aide who works privately with your child in the school setting. Some school districts employ an autism consultant who works with preschool staff to provide modifications that support your child's success in a mainstream setting. As with all educational services, exactly how your child's preschool experience is structured will vary depending on her needs, strengths, and challenges, as well as resources available in your community. During this time you may also choose to work with private practitioners (for example, behavioral specialists, speech pathologists, occupational therapists) to which your child's pediatrician refers you. Ideally, these practitioners will coordinate their services with those who work with your child in the school setting.

A PARENT'S STORY: NORA

When Nora's daughter Rory was first diagnosed with an autism spectrum disorder at 2 years of age, Nora and her family felt as if they were on their own. But they found a developmental pediatrician who was a wonderful resource.

After spending a few months with a private therapist, Rory went to an applied behavior analysis (ABA) class. But it was not a good fit for her.

"Another mother suggested a private tutor that she had been using, who was a preschool teacher for children with autism. We always say she turned out to be Rory's Annie Sullivan. That woman got her in line. Carolyn didn't give up. That first day Rory wanted her milk and Carolyn said, 'I'll give you your milk, but you have to say milk.' Rory screamed and cried and after about 20 minutes said 'milk.' It was incredible.

"Psychologists who evaluated Rory all agreed that she is very bright and capable of learning. She's known her alphabet since she was 2. She continued her private ABA lessons until she turned 3 and was sent to a private autism preschool that does 30 hours a week of ABA. She is now 5 and attending the same program but at the local elementary school. She also gets occupational therapy and speech therapy in school."

The bottom line to Nora's story: it will take time, energy, and patience, but to make progress, it's important to determine what therapy and therapists work best for you and your child.

Elementary School

Moving from preschool to an elementary school can be an exciting transition, but for children with ASDs, it can also be a challenging one. More people may be involved in your child's education, and there may be more transitions in a day than he had in preschool. Socializing with peers and interacting with more adults also becomes a bigger part of the day. Extracurricular activities may become part of the schedule, too.

According to law, children with disabilities must be placed in what is called the *least restrictive environment,* which requires school districts to educate children with ASDs in regular classrooms as much as possible. The goal is for the child to be taught in the most natural setting possible while still making progress. Some people call this mainstreaming, while others refer to it as integration or inclusion.

Why the push for the least restrictive environment? Experts believe that being in an inclusive setting allows children with ASDs to interact more frequently with people outside the special education environment. That means spending time with everyone from their typically developing peers, to support staff, to the custodial staff. Exposure to different groups allows for more social interactions, which can bolster a child's social skills, communication abilities, and confidence.

Of course, parents and others might not agree on the ideal classroom placement for a child with an ASD. Different school districts will have different policies about what works best. It's also possible for a child's needs to change over time. But wherever a child is placed, it's essential that there are supports in place to help him do his best. Possible classroom options include

- *Self-contained classroom.* The child is placed in a class only for children with disabilities.
- *Partial mainstreaming.* The child spends part of his day in a self-contained classroom and the other part in a regular classroom.
- *Full mainstreaming with support.* The child spends the entire day in a regular classroom with help from an aide.
- *Full mainstreaming without support.* The child spends the day in a regular classroom without an aide.

Integrating a child with an ASD into a classroom with his mainstream peers often requires some form of disability awareness training for the teachers and possibly for other students he will see during the day. Ideally, the classroom teacher will know about autism and will take the necessary steps to make the room a comfortable environment for your child. She should also take some time to talk to your family about what works best for your child. It's important that teachers assist your child as he transitions between activities and do what it takes to help him navigate social and communication challenges. For instance, the teacher may help identify peers who could be paired up with your child during lunch and recess so he receives support from classmates during 2 of the more social parts of the day.

Many children with ASDs also benefit from having the specialized therapies you read about in Chapter 4. For instance, your child may attend speech-language therapy to bolster his communication skills or occupational therapy to help with fine motor and self-care skills.

Some children may be encouraged to participate in a social skills group. A social skills group could help your child understand and practice his social interactions. Although the school setting is perfect for social skills training, it is also a difficult place to provide the amount and type of training that most children with ASDs may require. Studies on social skills training have found that most formal programs in schools may not be enough to make a difference in improving a child's social skills. That's why it may be important for parents to work on these skills with their child at home as peer interactions start to become more complex. Games that encourage cooperation, for instance, can teach kids how to get along better in group settings. Role-playing different social situations can help prepare your child for real-life situations in school. Presenting appropriate behaviors in the form of a story—also known as social stories—can be helpful as well. Explicit instructions for coping with tough situations, like how to deal with a bully, may be helpful. You can also use drawings to teach your child how to read moods, books to teach manners, and home videos to show how to behave in different situations.

For some children it is appropriate to have an aide or paraprofessional within the classroom. The aide can ensure that your child spends as much time in an inclusive setting as possible. Children at this level may also be given special academic accommodations to help them succeed. For instance, they may be allowed to do just the even-numbered problems on a math assignment. In this case, the child is able to show what he knows while not getting too frustrated doing a task that may increase anxiety and frustration. Your child may be eligible for adaptive physical education to increase participation through accommodations for social, communication, or motor difficulties. Some kids may be given a designated cooldown area if they experience increased anxiety during certain times of the day.

To enhance your child's elementary-level education, it's important to involve him in other activities like recreational programs, after-school clubs, and special interest groups. You may also want to enroll him in religious education, if that is important to you and your family. These groups not only tap into your child's interests but create additional opportunities for him to practice and hone his social and communication skills while participating in the life of his community. Your child's pediatrician and school team may be aware of extracurricular activities that are adapted for children with ASDs and other disabilities within your community. See Chapter 9 for more information on community-based activities for children with ASDs.

Middle School

The transition between elementary and middle school can be even more challenging for some children with ASDs. For starters, your child will now be switching classes every period instead of staying in one classroom for all subjects, which will place greater demand on his organization skills and ability to transition efficiently. He'll also be getting more time to complete longer-term assignments. Socially, your child may become more vulnerable to bullying as children become more aware of differences. His peers may choose to avoid him so they aren't associated with the "weird" kid. Any differences in his personal hygiene and habits may become more obvious as adolescents become increasingly self-conscious about their appearance. To make it even more challenging, early hormonal changes in puberty might make his emotions less predictable and more volatile, which can make it harder for him to regulate his fluctuating emotions. Your young teen may become moody, irritable, and hostile. He may have changes in eating and sleeping habits and may even lose interest in things that used to fascinate him.

Some children may require additional supports for these vulnerabilities, which should be spelled out in their IEP. Different schools will use different methods for providing that kind of support. In some schools, for instance, children with ASDs may be paired up with peer buddies who can help them navigate peer relationships. Extra effort from school staff and parents may be necessary to help a child stay organized. A child with an ASD may be placed in a supervised study hall staffed by a teacher, preferably with a special education background, who actively participates in helping the student organize assignments, directing the student's efforts to complete homework, and serving as a resource to assist the student in completing her work. The study hall teacher maintains communication with the student's regular teachers to make sure assignments are being recorded properly, completed, and handed in. Some districts may step up their efforts to communicate with parents.

Sexuality may become an issue at this age too. Important topics include sex education (including sex abuse education), self-care, hygiene, and intimate relationships. It's important to start these discussions early and regularly so when issues come up, it's possible to have a good, deep conversation that is at a level that your child understands. Helping children with ASDs and other developmental disabilities understand rules about touch, affection, and boundaries can be difficult. If your child has difficulty understanding social norms such as keeping private parts covered in public, you will need to discuss that with him. If you have trouble discussing these topics, take advantage of your child's pediatrician and professionals at the school, who can help you figure out the best ways to raise these issues and have meaningful conversations about them.

Social challenges may become more of an issue at this age, as peers begin to play a more important role. Some children may be overly sensitive to what their peers say or do, while others may be entirely indifferent. Others become prey for bullies.

With greater self-awareness, your child may begin to notice that he is different than others, so you should be prepared to discuss your child's diagnosis with him in an appropriate way. (See "Discussing an Autism Spectrum Disorder Diagnosis With Your Child" on page 106.)

To help your child navigate the social world of middle school, make sure to continue working with him on his social skills, especially if the school no longer has these programs available. Some schools have peer programs in which certain typical students are selected and assigned to interact with specific students with ASDs on a regular basis. If bullying is widespread, the district may conduct disability awareness training and school-wide anti-bullying programs for all students.

Remember that these are the years when your child may have more unstructured time outside of his school day. Use this as an opportunity to help her explore activities that appeal to his interests and goals, even those that may someday lead to a vocation or career. Look for ways to modify interests that may no longer seem age-appropriate and adapt them so they are. For instance, if a child loves to mold clay, consider enrolling him in a sculpting class. It's also important at this age to begin encouraging your child's independence and self-sufficiency. The more your child is able to do, the easier it will be for him later on to secure a job and live on his own.

High School

Entering high school is a big change for any child and marks the transition to adulthood. These are the years when you begin planning for life after school. Will your child go to college? Begin training for a job? Live on his own? While you are working through these important questions, it's essential that you continue to revisit your child's IEP so his educational program remains current and reflects his ongoing progress as well as any new concerns.

When your child starts high school, around the age of 14 years, it's important to begin the process of planning and setting long-term goals that will lead to development of a transition plan. Under IDEA law, a child's IEP is required to have a transition plan by the time he is 16 years old. The transition plan identifies the services your child will need to prepare for life after high school and describes his goals as he enters adulthood. The plan should reflect his personal desires and interests, while also discussing practical concerns such as employment options, continuing education, health care, long-term care, sibling support, and need for community, state, and federal resources.

To create a transition plan that promotes success after school, it's important to involve your teen as well as teachers, siblings, friends, and any other people who are intimately familiar with his skills, talents, and shortcomings. Conversations about the transition plan should

(continued on page 108)

DISCUSSING AN AUTISM SPECTRUM DISORDER DIAGNOSIS WITH YOUR CHILD

Parents may wonder about when and whether to tell their child about their autism spectrum disorder (ASD) diagnosis. Following are some commonly asked questions about discussing the diagnosis with a child with an ASD:

Should I tell my child about his diagnosis?

Parents may fear that finding out about the ASD will be hard on their child. Some children can initially find the news upsetting, especially if they are very sensitive to any suggestion that they are different from their peers. Many individuals with ASDs, however, have shared that learning they were on the autism spectrum suddenly made it clear why so many things had been difficult or why they had been treated differently. With increased awareness of ASDs, a diagnosis may also provide a reason for their behavior that they think other people might understand. For some, the diagnosis can take away the notion that past problems had all been the result of some personal failing; replacing this with the notion of a legitimate condition helps explain their challenges.

When should I tell my child that he has an ASD?

While it is important to tell an individual with an ASD about the diagnosis, there is no correct age or time to tell a child. A child's personality, abilities, and social awareness are all factors to consider in determining when he is ready for information about his diagnosis. For example, a parent may decide to talk about ASDs when the child begins asking questions such as, "Why am I different?"

Considering the potential effect of the information, how can a parent best explain to a child that he has an ASD?

- *Before you begin, assess what your child already knows and how well he will be able to take in a discussion about ASDs.*

- *Pitch the news at the right level.* Prepare to explain ASDs in terms your child can grasp. Too vague an explanation may not satisfy an inquisitive teenager, while too technical an explanation may confuse or frighten a child of any age. If circumstances lead to a very early first discussion about your child's differences, you may choose not to use the actual ASD label but discuss how some children learn differently or need help with certain things at school. Disclosing a more specific diagnosis can wait until your child's understanding grows.

- *Be positive.* When sharing news of a diagnosis with your child, you will want to keep things very positive. It's also a good idea to choose a time when you and your child are feeling good and when you won't be interrupted or distracted.

DISCUSSING AN AUTISM SPECTRUM DISORDER DIAGNOSIS WITH YOUR CHILD, CONTINUED

- *Tailor your explanation of ASDs to your child's own situation.* Start with the positive, then address the negative. It's important to tell the child that you love all the "good stuff" about him and you wouldn't ever want him to change. Undoubtedly, your child has been struggling in some areas because of ASD. It's OK to acknowledge these difficulties while emphasizing that it is not his fault that some things are difficult for him.

- *Describe ASDs as a different kind of disability.* If the child understands the concept of "disability," you might identify an ASD as just a different kind of disability. You can explain that people have a disability when something isn't working quite right and they need extra help because of it. People with ASDs, for example, might need extra help in understanding others and making friends. It may be helpful to illustrate how all children learn differently by giving examples of children they know who get extra help in other areas.

- *Stress that you'll be there.* You should emphasize that you and other family members, teachers, and therapists are going to stick by the child, supporting him as he works on things that are hard for him. You'll encourage him when it's tough and cheer when he has a success. You'll celebrate the good stuff while helping with the not-so-good stuff.

- *Let the child know there are a lot of other people with ASDs.* Your child is definitely not alone, and it is important to let him know this. Your child may be interested in and benefit from meeting others with ASDs.

- *Raise your child's awareness.* Even before you discuss your child's diagnosis with him, it may be helpful to read books in which characters have ASDs and other disabilities and watch shows with your child in which characters have disabilities so that awareness of individual differences is presented gradually and as part of everyday life.

Sharing information about ASDs in a positive, matter-of-fact, and age-appropriate way helps set the stage for a child's ability to understand, accept, and adapt to the reality of an ASD in his life. Keep in mind that the whole concept of "having an ASD" is a lot to take in. It's going to be a process that takes some time, with new questions asked and deeper understanding gained as a child matures.

For additional information on discussing ASDs with your child, see Appendix A. Make sure your pediatrician knows about your questions and concerns, and share the information you find in your research. You might ask about a referral to a mental health professional for some additional therapy for your child and for some ongoing parent coaching as well. Remember, you and your pediatrician are partners in your child's health.

Adapted with permission of Kennedy Krieger Institute, Baltimore, MD. This information appeared originally at www.iancommunity. org/cs/articles/telling_a_child_about_his_asd.

include questions that assess academic skills (reading, math, and writing) and personal skills (social strengths, interests, reliability) such as

- What does your teen like to do?
- What are his dreams, goals, and interests in terms of work?
- What are his strengths? What can he do?
- What are some areas that he still needs to explore and learn?
- What does he need to learn to reach his goals?
- What are some future education goals?
- How do you and your teen feel about him getting a job?
- Where are some viable places for employment?
- What kinds of transportation does he have available to him?
- Where will he live?
- What kind of health insurance will your teen have down the road?
- Does he require supports in developing friendships?
- Is he well known in the community?
- Does he need help structuring his recreation time?
- What hobbies and interests does he have?

When formulating your teen's goals, it's important to think about his learning skills, communication skills, and ability to deal with sensory input. Is he a slow learner? Does he have a strategy for communicating that is effective, even if he doesn't speak clearly? Is he able to deal with new sights, sounds, and smells that he may confront in the community or workplace?

In considering any future employment opportunities, it's important to consider what kinds of job training or postsecondary education your teen will want. Some teens may have very specific goals in mind that may require more long-term planning. Your current school district may work with agencies and community partners to help your teen secure the support and training he will need. It's also important to know that several colleges and universities now offer programs geared specifically to students who have ASDs and other disabilities.

Difficulties in School

School can be a wonderful place for learning, friendships, and honing the life skills that any child will need to succeed. But for some children it can also be a challenging place, filled with stress, social anxieties, and performance concerns. These problems may be more commonly experienced by children who have ASDs.

Challenging Behaviors

As anyone who has ever gone through school knows, good behavior is critical to a student's academic performance. But children with ASDs may struggle with behaviors that are counterproductive to their progress and even disruptive to other students.

If your child is having behavioral problems, a team of professionals may do a functional behavioral analysis, or FBA. As you may recall, an FBA identifies the antecedents and consequences surrounding a specific behavior and creates a plan for intervening that will alter the behavior, as well as ways to gauge whether the intervention is working. The IEP team can arrange for the FBA. In fact, IDEA law requires that an FBA be done when a child is having behavior problems.

The process begins with identifying the problem behavior in clear, concrete terms. For instance, rather than say that "Johnny is rude," an FBA would say, "Johnny shoves, kicks, and hits other children during transition time." The description should be expressed in specific, observable, and measurable terms.

Next, you need to create a plan to collect data. Gathering data may be done in 1 of 2 ways, directly or indirectly. Collecting data directly involves observing circumstances surrounding the problem behavior. Does the problem occur just before lunch when the child may be hungry? Does it arise whenever she's in a crowded auditorium? Is she more apt to act out when new lessons are being taught? Are behaviors preceded by the same incidents each time? Find out how often the problem behavior occurs and in what kind of intervals. Doing an antecedent, behavior, consequence (ABC) observation form can help too. Each time a child misbehaves, record the inappropriate behavior and what happened just before it, which are the *antecedents*. Then record what happens after it, which are the *consequences* of that behavior. Record only what you see and hear without interpreting the behavior.

Gathering data may also be done indirectly using student records, questionnaires, or checklists to see how others perceive the behavior. It may involve interviews with other staff members to find out who's present when the problem behavior occurs, when and where it tends to happen, and what's happening before and after the behavior. This information should be collected from several sources including teachers, counselors, and after-school supervisors.

After a few days, you should begin to see a pattern that links the child's behavior to her environment. You'll be able to predict events that lead to the problem behavior and identify consequences that perpetuate it. Remember, most problem behaviors serve a purpose and are done to attain something or avoid something.

In addition, it is critical to understand that certain aspects of a child's ASD may be the underlying cause of a behavior. For example, a child with oversensitive hearing may act out during a noisy gym class. So an intervention needs to consider sensory and biological problems that manifest as a result of the ASD.

The next step is to develop and implement a behavioral intervention plan (BIP). Children generally respond better to methods that are positive and which encourage and teach appropriate, alternative behaviors. You might try modifying the physical environment, adjusting the curriculum, or changing antecedents or consequences for the problem behavior. It's also helpful to teach a more acceptable behavior that serves the same purpose.

Once you implement the plan, make sure to monitor the child's progress over time. If interventions aren't working, you may need to go back and devise a new strategy.

If a behavioral problem becomes so severe that teachers recommend a child be expelled or moved to a different setting for 10 days or longer, your child may be given a manifestation determination hearing to determine if the behavior was related to the child's disability. The manifestation review is conducted by the school district, parent, and other members of the IEP team within 10 days of the suspension or change in placement. If the behavior was related to the disability, the child is returned to the classroom. The IEP team must then do an FBA and BIP within 10 days of the manifestation determination, or modify the existing one to address the problem behavior.

Stress and the Rage Cycle

Children who have ASDs are prone to anxiety and stress. In fact, anxiety disorders are one of the most common coexisting medical conditions in children with ASDs. Children with ASDs may be thrust into confusing social situations that are difficult for them to understand or handle. Their sometimes rigid rules about injustice and their innate emotional vulnerability make it difficult for them to manage certain events that other children may readily dismiss. As a result, they may experience a lot of stress, which causes them to withdraw or become preoccupied with obsessions and thoughts. They may also become hyperactive, aggressive, and difficult. To compound the situation, many of these children have difficulty recognizing the stress they feel and see no problem with their behaviors.

Experts like Brenda Smith Myles, PhD, have called the sequence of events around stress the *rage cycle.* In the right setting with the right triggers, almost all of us can become entrapped in a rage cycle. But most children with typical development create strategies for dealing with situations that make them angry. And certainly by adulthood, most of us can better handle upsetting stressors.

Children with ASDs, however, are more vulnerable to outbursts because they are naturally more prone to anxiety and have less self-awareness. It's important to understand that the meltdown occurs for a reason—there is often a reason for or cause of the angry behavior. That's why FBAs are so important to understanding the behavior of a child with an ASD. Exploding into a tantrum is not something a child wants to do, but it's often the only way the child can express himself because his communication skills are inadequate.

Parents and teachers can help reduce the child's anxiety and stress by understanding the rage cycle and deploying strategies that help children manage their stress. (It's also why it's so important to improve your child's understanding of social situations, arm him with the skills for living and working in a world with other people, and master communication skills that will help him express himself.) The rage cycle has 3 distinct phases—rumbling, meltdown or rage, and recovery. Early in the cycle, there are distinct strategies for preventing or decreasing the problem behavior.

Rumbling

The rage cycle begins with the rumbling stage. At this point, you may notice some minor behavioral changes that have little to do with the impending meltdown. The child may clear his throat, lower his voice, tense his muscles, or tap his feet. Facial expressions may give away feelings of unhappiness. Other behaviors may be more obvious. The child may withdraw physically or emotionally from what's going on around him, or he may lash out physically or verbally at someone else. If it's happening in a classroom, the child may attempt to engage in a power struggle with the teacher.

Nipping the problem at the rumbling stage is critical to preventing a meltdown, and teachers and parents have several strategies at their disposal. These include

- *Removing the child.* If the problem occurs in school, the teacher can send the child on an errand. If it's happening at home, the parent can ask the child to retrieve an object. The brief absence can help the child regain his calm so that when he comes back, the problem has usually lessened.
- *Moving closer to the child.* When a teacher senses a child's distress, she can simply walk over and be near the child. Parents can do the same. Simply putting yourself in close proximity to the child can lessen his stress without disrupting other students.
- *Signaling the child.* A teacher who has a child prone to rage can work out a signal in advance that lets the child know she is aware of the situation. Making the signal, which can be as simple as tapping the desk or putting a pencil behind her ear, can be reassuring to the child and may be used just before removing the child from the situation.
- *Supporting his routine.* A child with an ASD may rely on predictability. Having a visual schedule of events in the day can make him feel safe and ease his stress. It also helps to let him know ahead of time about any schedule changes.
- *Redirecting.* Shifting the child's attention to something other than what's upsetting him can often help reduce his stress. While it's OK to postpone a new activity in some situations, in others he may need to be redirected immediately. The child may also be redirected to a pre-rehearsed calming sequence or use relaxation techniques that have been practiced with a therapist beforehand.

- *Giving him a safe place to go.* Some experts call this a home base, a place where the child can go to escape stress. The safe place should have minimal distractions, and activities in the area should be soothing, not stimulating. In school, there could be a safe place in the classroom, such as a table in the corner, and when that is not enough, another safe haven outside the classroom might be the counselor's office. At home, it might be the child's bedroom. Wherever it is, the safe place should be viewed as a positive retreat, not an area used for time-outs or special play. It might also be used as a place for the child to regroup during the recovery phase of the rage cycle.
- *Acknowledging difficulties.* When the rumbling stage is triggered by a challenging task, it can sometimes help to simply acknowledge that the task is hard and then encourage the child to proceed anyway. A simple verbal acknowledgment may be enough to prevent the child from having a tantrum.
- *Walking, not talking.* Taking a short, silent stroll with a distraught child can sometimes help soothe a child on the brink of a meltdown. The accompanying adult should say nothing, while allowing the child to vent any upsetting emotions without consequence.

As you can see, these strategies are not difficult to do and are, in fact, sometimes quite simple. But the effect they have on a child's impending tantrum can be huge. The key is knowing which one to use in which situation and not allowing yourself to become part of the struggle. It's also important to avoid certain behaviors that can escalate the child's rage and almost guarantee a meltdown. These include raising your voice, focusing on who's right, preaching, being sarcastic, using physical force, acting superior, pleading, bribing, and insisting on having the last word. An adult should also never attack the child's character, make unsubstantiated accusations, compare the child to others, or insult or humiliate the child.

Meltdown/Rage

If you aren't able to diffuse the situation in the rumbling stage, the child will go into the meltdown or rage stage. Behavior at this point is erratic and out of control. The child no longer has the ability to process information and may be quite physically aggressive—hitting, kicking, and biting—or verbally abusive. He may hurt himself or others or damage property. In some cases, the child may completely withdraw. Most times, the meltdown will have to run its course.

The focus at this point should be the safety of the child, his classmates, and adults. It's also important to try and help the child regain some semblance of control by whisking him off to his safe place or enlisting the help of other people on the school staff. Ideally, a plan should be in place before a tantrum occurs so staff and teachers are fully prepared.

Recovery

When the tantrum subsides, the child may feel badly about what's happened. He may also not fully remember what has just occurred. He remains fragile and may need time to rest before rejoining the class. The recovery period is not the time to teach the child new lessons or lecture on what has just occurred. Rather, the best thing to do is to help the child simply fall back into the routine of the class. A teacher can do this best by leading the child to a task he enjoys and does well.

By understanding the stages of the rage cycle, teachers and parents alike can help a child with an ASD deal with stress and prevent bad situations from escalating into full-blown tantrums. It often takes time to figure out which strategies work best with each child and with which situation. Over time and with practice, the child may even learn to generalize strategies that work best and be able to apply them to other stressful situations.

Understanding and using educational services and strategies are important to help your child feel successful in a school setting. In some cases, though, strategies that involve medications may also be helpful. In the following chapter we'll review the most common medications prescribed for children with ASDs and factors to consider when evaluating this option.

Autism Champion: Brenda Smith Myles, PhD

Brenda Smith Myles, PhD, has always spent time with children on the autism spectrum—one of her first playmates had autism, though Dr Myles was never told so. As a graduate student, she still remembers a little boy who threw a tantrum and stormed out of the room when she didn't draw a dinosaur correctly. "I ran after him, and from that moment on, I was intrigued, challenged, and in love with autism," she says.

That was back in 1982 when autism was less well known. As a graduate student in special education, Dr Myles was the associate director of a clinic at the University of Kansas that trained master's students how to work with children who had learning disabilities and behavioral challenges. None of them had been diagnosed, but Dr Myles learned to recognize these students as having high-functioning autism. "Every place I turned, it seemed I should be working with kids with autism and their families," she says.

Which is exactly what Dr Myles did. She wrote the first federal grant in the country that created a master's program in Asperger syndrome at the University of Kansas. She also went on to write more than 150 books and articles on autism spectrum disorders (ASDs), including *Asperger Syndrome and Difficult Moments: Practical Solutions for Tantrums, Rage, and Meltdowns,* a book she wrote in 5 days with her colleague Jack Southwick.

It was Dr Myles who coined the term *rage cycle,* which describes the pattern of behaviors that result in the tantrums that are common in children with ASDs. "Originally, we were going to call the book *Asperger Syndrome and Rage,* but parents wouldn't say it was rage," Dr Myles recalls. "So we changed it to 'difficult moments.' Parents influence everything I do."

Dr Myles, who is a parent to a typically developing 18-year-old, has garnered numerous accolades for her efforts. In a survey by the University of Texas, she was named the second most productive applied researcher in ASDs in the world. She is currently a consultant with the Ziggurat Group, an organization that provides assessment, consultation, and training to benefit individuals with ASDs across the life span. Dr Myles regards the diagnosis and program planning assessment conducted by the Ziggurat Group interdisciplinary team as the best in the nation. She lectures globally about ASDs and has given more than 500 presentations. "There are many countries doing a nice job with individuals on the spectrum," she says. "But I think the US is certainly rising to meet their needs."

Her goal now is to encourage more collaboration so that individual institutions, states, and even countries aren't always reinventing the wheel. For instance, she recently helped create standards for teachers of children with ASDs, which were just accepted by the National Council for Accreditation of Teacher Education. "It's all about bringing organizations and people together to collaborate and making sure individuals with autism reach their potential," she says. "I know that sounds idealistic, but I am from Kansas—a place where anything can happen. Just ask Dorothy."

CHAPTER 6

When Other Therapies Aren't Enough: The Role of Medication

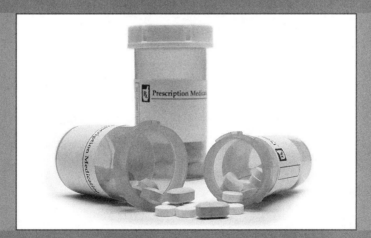

Medications may help many conditions, but they are not the main treatment for children with autism spectrum disorders (ASDs). They do not directly target the social skill and language deficits that are at the core of ASDs. Still, medications may help address other medical conditions that are common in children with ASDs such as sleep problems, gastrointestinal (GI) conditions, and seizures. They may also be considered in addition to behavioral therapy for certain problems such as hyperactivity, impulsivity, inattention, irritability, anxiety, aggression, self-injury, and repetitive behaviors, especially if they disrupt your child's learning, socializing, health, safety, or quality of life. Medications can be an option if behavioral treatments alone are not sufficient or as a way to help support other therapies.

In this chapter, we'll look at the most common medications prescribed for children with ASDs. We'll also look at factors to consider when making a decision about starting a medication for your child.

Is Medication Warranted?

Although medications are not the first line of therapy for children with ASDs, recent surveys show that approximately 45% to 50% of children and adolescents with ASDs are treated with medications to address behavioral problems. These drugs are more likely to be used in older children and in those with fewer adaptive skills, less social awareness, and more challenging behaviors. We will discuss some of these drugs later in this chapter.

So if medications aren't the primary treatment for ASDs, why are so many children taking them? Many children with ASDs have accompanying psychiatric conditions, such as anxiety, depression, or mood instability, that when left untreated, interfere with significant aspects of their lives. Treating these associated psychiatric conditions makes it possible for children with ASDs to function at a higher level than they otherwise would. It also may enable them to more successfully navigate the demands of their daily routines. In the past it was thought that some of these conditions, such as anxiety and attention-deficit/hyperactivity disorder (ADHD), were simply part of autism. We now know that children with ASDs are more likely than the general population to have other psychiatric conditions and that these conditions are treatable.

Even so, the decision to start medication for a child with an ASD is not something done lightly. Here are some things you should do before moving in this direction.

- Before starting your child on any drug, it's important to work with your pediatrician to see if there is a medical condition that may be the underlying cause of your child's behavior problems. For example, a child with an ASD and constipation may communicate her discomfort by yelling, screaming, or even hitting if she has difficulty verbally communicating with her caregivers. Many medical issues that cause pain or distress, such as infections, allergies, GI disorders, or dental issues, may increase behavioral problems in children with ASDs. Likewise, children who are not sleeping well at night are more prone to daytime irritability. Even something as simple as an ear infection may cause a child to behave disruptively.

- Look at what else is going on in her life. It's important to consider that changes in the environment may be causing the problematic behavior. Be on the lookout for new demands on your child, changes in her routine, or new transitions, all of which may upset her. The arrival of a new teacher at school, for example, may be causing your child to lose sleep, which in turn might make her more prone to repetitive behaviors.

- Do a thorough assessment of the problem behavior. Identify how long it has been going on and how long each episode lasts. Are there certain factors or situations that seem to trigger it? How has the problem behavior changed over time? Is it increasing, decreasing, or somewhat stable? Determine how big of an effect it is having on your child. Is it affecting her ability to learn? Is it hindering academic progress, affecting her relations with peers, or putting her or others at risk of harm? Understanding the ABCs of the behavior—*a*ntecedent, *b*ehavior, and *c*onsequence (as described in Chapter 4)—is also very helpful.

- Always consider behavioral strategies first before thinking about medications. In many instances, a medication may be used to supplement a behavioral intervention. The exception might be if your child's safety or the safety of others is at risk.

Following are some health conditions or behavioral problems common in children with ASDs that may make you consider, or may in fact require, using medication:

Seizures

When abnormal or excessive electrical impulses occur in the brain, your child may have a *seizure*. During a seizure, neurons in the brain may fire faster, more suddenly, and more out of sequence than normal. The abnormal brain activity may cause changes in physical movement, sensation, or behavior. Seizures that occur repeatedly over time without an underlying illness such as a fever or brain injury are known as *epilepsy*. Approximately 25% of all people with ASDs may have a seizure during their lifetime. Seizures are more common in children who have intellectual disabilities, genetic conditions, or problems with motor skills. The onset of seizures is most common in children before the age of 5 years and during adolescence.

During a seizure, muscles may stiffen up or become completely relaxed. Some seizures involve the entire body, whereas others only involve one part of the body, such as the face, a limb, or one side. A child having a seizure may have rapid, violent movements and even lose consciousness. Less dramatic seizures may consist of momentary lapses of attention that can cause a blank stare for a few moments. Some seizures are so subtle that they go unnoticed.

If your doctor suspects your child is having seizures, she may do an electroencephalogram (EEG), a test that records electrical activity in the brain. Though an EEG is generally not recommended as part of the routine evaluation for ASDs, doctors may recommend them for symptoms that suggest seizures. Some children may have abnormalities on their EEGs without having seizures. Some studies have shown that EEG abnormalities are more common in children who have autistic regression (see Chapter 3).

Treating children who have ASDs with epilepsy is the same as it is in other children with epilepsy and involves antiseizure medication. There are numerous medicines in this category; some of the most common include phenobarbital, phenytoin (Dilantin), carbamazepine (Tegretol), valproic acid (Depakote), oxcarbazepine (Trileptal), lamotrigine (Lamictal), and levetiracetam (Keppra). Antiseizure medications can have serious side effects, and your child should be closely monitored. But once you find the proper dosage for your child, the number of seizures can usually be reduced, although not always completely controlled. Your child may need periodic blood tests after he starts a medication to make sure there is enough in his system and to monitor for side effects. He also may need occasional EEGs to see how well the medicine is working. Medication is usually weaned gradually after he has had no seizures for a year or two. In some cases, though, seizures may persist indefinitely, or it may take longer for a child to cease having seizures. A child may, in fact, have to resume medication or take medication for a longer period. Some antiseizure medicines are also used as mood stabilizers.

Tics

Some children with ASDs have *tics,* or brief, involuntary movements and sounds, which are also the defining symptoms of a neurologic condition called Tourette syndrome. A child with an ASD may have tics or tic-like behavior but not meet the strict diagnosis of Tourette syndrome. The 2 conditions have a lot in common including echolalia, obsessive-compulsive behaviors, and abnormal motor behaviors. Some experts believe that the same brain abnormalities in ASDs also exist in Tourette syndrome. Medications used to treat tics include alpha-2 agonists (such as clonidine and guanfacine) and others such as atypical antipsychotics.

Gastrointestinal Problems

Many children with ASDs experience GI issues such as chronic constipation, abdominal pain, or diarrhea. In fact, studies report that from 9% to 70% or more of children with ASDs have GI problems.

Some children with pain or discomfort from GI issues may act out by hurting themselves, throwing tantrums, or behaving aggressively. Many will have trouble sleeping. Gastrointestinal problems may also delay toilet training in some children with ASDs.

Treating GI issues will vary, depending on the problem. Children with constipation, for instance, may require stool softeners. Those who have gastroesophageal reflux disease may benefit from a medication like ranitidine (Zantac) to reduce acid and heartburn. Children with lactose intolerance benefit from a lactose-free diet. For more information about these treatments, see Chapter 7.

A PARENT'S STORY: RONNY

"From the time CJ was 6 months to the age of 3, he has had diarrhea. Doctors kept telling us it wasn't uncommon in kids with autism. But we finally took him to a GI doctor. An x-ray showed he had an obstruction in his bowels.

"The doctor suggested he take MiraLax [polyethylene glycol], an over-the-counter laxative. Now he takes 1 scoop every day in his morning drink. Every 2 weeks, he takes 4 scoops throughout his day. The MiraLax continually breaks down the feces, and CJ can have normal bowel movements."

Sleep Disturbances

Many children experience sleep challenges at one time or another. In fact, 3% of all visits to pediatricians are to address sleep problems. But the problem is greater in children with ASDs, with about 30% to 75% having sleep difficulties.

There are many different causes of sleep problems in children with ASDs. Primary sleep disorders, such as obstructive sleep apnea, restless legs syndrome, and delayed sleep phase syndrome, have been reported in children with ASDs. Additionally, the core behaviors associated with ASDs may predispose children with ASDs to behaviorally based sleep disorders. Elements related to bedtime routines and the sleep environment, such as viewing television or playing video games close to bedtime, drinking caffeinated beverages, or a having a room that is too warm, loud, or lit, may lead to sleep difficulties. Lastly, medical and psychiatric disorders, such as epilepsy, gastroesophageal reflux, anxiety, and depression, may be the cause of a child's sleep problem. Table 6-1 has more information about common sleep problems in children with ASDs.

The 2 most common types of sleep problems are trouble getting to sleep and waking up at night. For children with ASDs, getting to sleep can be difficult because of hyperactivity, anxiety, and poorly regulated sleep-wake cycles. Some children may be going to bed too early or before they're in a fully relaxed state.

TABLE 6-1. COMMON SLEEP PROBLEMS IN CHILDREN WITH AUTISM SPECTRUM DISORDERS	
Condition	**Description**
Obstructive sleep apnea	Occurs when there is a blockage (sometimes from enlarged tonsils or adenoid) that does not allow air to adequately enter into the lungs. Symptoms include loud snoring, pauses in breathing or gasping breaths, difficulty waking in the morning, and daytime sleepiness or irritability.
Restless legs syndrome	Restless legs syndrome involves an urge to move the legs or an uncomfortable sensation in the legs that typically occurs at bedtime. It is worse at rest and is relieved by movement. Children may complain of leg pain, have difficulty finding a comfortable position to fall asleep, or be restless sleepers.
Delayed sleep phase syndrome	A disorder of sleep-wake cycles (circadian rhythm) in which the individual has difficulty falling asleep and may often have difficulty waking up the next morning. This condition may be more common in children with autism spectrum disorders because of insufficient melatonin production.

Some children wake up in the middle of the night and can't get back to sleep. These children may not have mastered the self-soothing techniques that help them drift off again when they awaken in the middle of the night during normal cycles of sleep. Any attention they receive during night awakenings, such as snacks or companionship, can worsen difficulties because children with ASDs may become dependent on these routines to fall back asleep. Still others may be battling physical discomfort such as restless legs or acid reflux.

Identifying the cause of a sleep problem requires a physical examination and a thorough review of your child's health history. It also involves doing a detailed report about your child's nightly bedtime routine, nighttime awakenings, and how you respond to those awakenings. What does your child do before bed every night and how long does it take for her to fall asleep? Does she snore, or is she a restless sleeper? Where does your child sleep and with whom? What foods does she eat close to bedtime, if any? Does your child watch television before bed? Do you lie down with her? What have you done to try and solve the problem?

All of this information is important for understanding your child's sleep challenges and providing the right treatment. Keeping a sleep diary for 2 weeks to determine the severity of the problem is also helpful. Occasionally, more tests may be needed. For example, if your pediatrician suspects a primary sleep disorder, he may recommend a referral to a sleep medicine specialist or arrange for a sleep study (also called polysomnography). A sleep study involves your child staying overnight in a sleep laboratory attached to monitoring equipment. The information from this study will be used by your pediatrician or sleep specialist to better understand the cause and severity of your child's sleep problem.

Before Medications: Importance of Sleep Hygiene and Behavioral Treatments

Sleep Hygiene

No matter what the cause of your child's sleep problem, treatment always begins with good sleep hygiene, or habits that support healthy sleep. Your child's sleep environment should be cool, with as little light and sound as possible. Healthy daytime habits include regular physical activity and limiting caffeinated beverages and naps. Healthy evening habits include limiting media exposure (video games, television, and computer) and having predictable bedtime routines. Good sleep hygiene is the first step in treating any sleep problems and sometimes works by itself to help such problems. If not, other steps may be needed.

Behavioral Treatments

Many types of sleep problems will respond to behavioral treatments. One technique, known as graduated extinction, may be helpful for difficulty falling asleep and night awakenings.

Graduated extinction is basically planning an exit from your child's room at bedtime or after a nighttime awakening. It does mean that you will ignore any disruptive behavior by not returning to the room for a predetermined amount of time. If done consistently, it can be effective, even with children with ASDs and other developmental disabilities. The process begins at bedtime when you say "good night" and give your child some praise for going to bed on his own. After that, you will check on your child at predetermined intervals and ignore any protests from your child in between these checks. Checks should be brief glances into the bedroom. If your child is still up, reassure yourself that he is OK but encourage him to go to sleep, then leave the room quickly without engaging him.

As the nights go on, lengthen the time between checks. Some parents decide to go in for their first check after 5 minutes, then over successive nights lengthen the interval of time between checks by a minute or even more. Before starting, make sure that all caregivers agree to adhere to the plan. Set a goal to do graduated extinction for a period of time, say 2 to 3 weeks. You should expect that your child's protest may reach a fevered pitch around days 2 or 3 (called the extinction burst) but if you stick with it, improvements should be obvious by the end of the first week.

Depending on your child's sleep patterns and habits, you may also want to try other behavioral strategies. If your child is simply not tired at bedtime, temporarily moving bedtime later until he's really tired, for instance, may help. Over time, as he becomes more successful at falling asleep, you can gradually move up his bedtime to an earlier hour. If you've been sleeping with your child to help him doze off, you might try moving further away from your child until he is finally able to fall asleep on his own in his own room. This may help him fall back to sleep on his own if he awakens at night.

Although difficult for some families, a technique known as scheduled awakenings may help alleviate frequent night awakenings. If your child awakens during the night at about the same time, you may want to try gently rousing your child (just get his eyes to open for a few seconds) 15 minutes before the time he usually awakens. After a number of nights of this, wait to see if he sleeps through the problem time. If so, you may have helped to reset his sleep cycle.

If behavioral strategies and improved sleep hygiene don't work, you may want to make an appointment with your child's pediatrician to discuss other treatments. The evidence for using medication to manage sleep disturbances in children with ASDs is limited. Except as otherwise noted, more studies are needed to establish the effectiveness of these medications for children with ASDs. Medications that can help manage sleep disturbances include the following:

- *Melatonin.* The body naturally produces this hormone, which helps regulate sleep cycles. A number of studies have shown that children with ASDs may make less melatonin than typically developing peers. Taking supplemental melatonin an hour before bedtime can help establish a normal sleep-wake cycle and help your child get to sleep. Melatonin is typically not long-acting, so it is mainly useful for children who have trouble falling asleep; it is less effective for those who have problems waking at night. Side effects include nightmares and nighttime waking. Several high-quality studies have demonstrated that melatonin can be effective in helping children with ASDs and sleep problems fall asleep sooner and have a longer total sleep time.

- *Clonidine* (Catapres, Kapvay). Clonidine is in a class of medications called centrally acting alpha-2 agonist agents, which are used to treat high blood pressure. It decreases heart rate and relaxes the blood vessels so that blood can flow more easily. Used off-label—meaning it's being used for purposes beyond what the US Food and Drug Administration (FDA) has approved it for—clonidine may help children with ASDs reduce hyperactivity, impulsivity, aggression, and tics while improving attention. If your child is prescribed clonidine, your pediatrician will monitor his blood pressure. The main side effect of clonidine is drowsiness because it may be used to help children with ASDs fall and stay asleep. For that reason, it may be given at night as a sleep aid. Morning drowsiness can be a side effect.

- *Guanfacine* (Tenex, Intuniv). Guanfacine is similar to clonidine, as it is also used to treat high blood pressure. It is used for the same purposes as clonidine (to reduce hyperactivity and impulsivity) but may be less sedating than clonidine. For this reason, it may not be used as commonly as clonidine for sleep, but it is used by some physicians occasionally for sleep issues.

- *Diphenhydramine* (Benadryl). Diphenhydramine is an antihistamine with sedating effects. Although commonly used for sleep problems, diphenhydramine has not been well studied as a sleep medicine. While it may be safe and effective for short-term insomnia, it may cause dry mouth, excitation, next-day drowsiness, as well as rebound insomnia (when sleep worsens after treatment ends).

- *Hydroxyzine* (Atarax, Vistaril). Hydroxyzine is an older antihistamine that also has a sedating effect. Unlike diphenhydramine, a prescription is required for hydroxyzine. It can cause the same side effects as diphenhydramine. While diphenhydramine and hydroxyzine can help with sleep because both have sedation as side effects, neither has been well studied specifically as a sleep aid for children.

- *Mirtazapine* (Remeron). This is a medicine used as an antidepressant in adults that affects the neurotransmitter (chemical signal in the brain) serotonin. Because it induces sleep, mirtazapine is often prescribed for children with sleep difficulties; it has not been studied specifically as a sleep aid in children with ASDs. It may also help with anxiety and mood. Side effects include excessive sedation, dry mouth, weight gain, and constipation.

- *Trazodone* (Desyrel). Trazodone is also used to treat depression in adults and affects serotonin. Because of its sedative properties, it has been used in low doses to induce sleep in children. Excessive sedation, dry mouth, nausea, and blurred vision may be side effects. Very rarely, a condition known as priapism—a painful, sustained erection—has been reported in boys and men. Although occasionally used to address sleep problems, there are no studies on using trazodone for sleep problems in children with ASDs.

Remember: Even if you do give your child a medication to address his sleep problems, it's still important to use behavioral interventions to help your child into a good sleep pattern.

WHAT'S GOOD SLEEP HYGIENE?

Sometimes, good sleep hygiene, or habits that support healthy sleep, is all it takes to overcome sleep difficulties in your child. Here's what you need to do.

- Have your child go to bed and get up at the same time every day, even on weekends.

- Create a relaxing routine in the hour or so leading up to bedtime.

- Make sure your child's bedroom is conducive to sleep, which means the room is quiet, cool, and dark and does not have a television, computer, or other electronics.

- Do not engage your child in play at bedtime or use bedtime as a punishment.

- Teach your child to fall asleep in her own bed, alone.

- Teach your child to fall asleep in conditions that will help her back to sleep if she awakens in the middle of the night.

Treating Psychiatric Conditions

It's not unusual for children who have ASDs to be treated with psychopharmacologic medications, drugs that affect the chemistry of the brain, to improve neurobehavioral functioning. Children who have ASDs are vulnerable to neurobehavioral problems that may meet criteria for other psychiatric conditions. But it's often difficult to separate autism from these other conditions. For instance, children who have ASDs may be naturally more anxious and yet not be labeled as having generalized anxiety disorder. Others may be hyperactive and impulsive and yet not be labeled as having ADHD. Whether there should be a separate diagnosis or not is a topic of debate among professionals in the field; the important point is that numerous children with ASDs may benefit from psychopharmacologic medication to improve neurologically based behaviors that are interfering with their ability to function and their quality of life.

The specific disorders that may exist with ASDs are

- *Generalized anxiety disorder.* Generalized anxiety disorder is excessive and uncontrollable worry about everyday matters. The worrying is disproportionate to the actual event and in some cases, may begin to interfere with daily functioning.
- *Major depression.* As many as 1 in 13 adolescents in the general population suffers from major depression, which can be tricky to diagnose in children. This disorder involves ongoing sadness, discouragement, loss of self-worth, and loss of interest in usual activities. Some children won't seem sad at all but may instead act out by misbehaving and getting in trouble.
- *Bipolar disorder.* Previously known as manic depression, people with bipolar disorder have extreme mood swings that alternate between euphoric highs and despairing lows. In children, bipolar disorder may be seen as agitation with explosive behavior.
- *Obsessive-compulsive disorder (OCD).* People who have OCD become consumed with repeating certain rituals and behaviors and may become obsessed with certain thoughts.
- *Attention-deficit/hyperactivity disorder.* This is a childhood disorder characterized by hyperactivity, impulsivity, and difficulty paying attention. It occurs in approximately 7% of all children and may be more common in children with ASDs.

Common Medications for Psychiatric Disorders

Many of the conditions described in this chapter are commonly treated with medication from the categories included in Table 6-2.

TABLE 6-2. POSSIBLE MEDICATION FOR CHILDREN WITH AUTISM SPECTRUM DISORDERS	
Coexisting Condition	**Medication Considerations**
Obsessive-compulsive disorder	SSRIs: fluoxetine[a] (Prozac), fluvoxamine[a] (Luvox), citalopram (Celexa), escitalopram (Lexapro), paroxetine (Paxil), sertraline (Zoloft) Atypical antipsychotic agents: risperidone[a] (Risperdal), aripiprazole[a] (Abilify), olanzapine (Zyprexa), quetiapine (Seroquel), ziprasidone (Geodon) Valproic acid[a] (Depakene, Depakote)
Attention-deficit/hyperactivity disorder	Stimulants: methylphenidate[a] (Ritalin, Ritalin LA, Methylin, Focalin, Focalin XR, Concerta, Metadate CD, Daytrana), dextroamphetamine (Dexedrine), lisdexamfetamine (Vyvanse), mixed amphetamine salts (Adderall, Adderall XR) Alpha-2 agonists: clonidine[a] (Catapres, Kapvay), guanfacine (Tenex, Intuniv) Atomoxetine[a] (Strattera) Atypical antipsychotic agents: risperidone[a] (Risperdal), aripiprazole[a] (Abilify), olanzapine[a] (Zyprexa), quetiapine (Seroquel), ziprasidone (Geodon)
Intermittent explosive disorder (aggression, irritability, self-injury)	Atypical antipsychotic agents: risperidone[a] (Risperdal), aripiprazole[a] (Abilify), olanzapine (Zyprexa), quetiapine (Seroquel), ziprasidone (Geodon) Alpha-2 agonists: clonidine[a] (Catapres, Kapvay), guanfacine (Tenex, Intuniv) Anticonvulsant mood stabilizers: valproic acid[a] (Depakene, Depakote), levetiracetam (Keppra), topiramate (Topamax) SSRIs: fluoxetine[a] (Prozac), fluvoxamine[a] (Luvox), citalopram (Celexa), escitalopram (Lexapro), paroxetine (Paxil), sertraline (Zoloft) Beta blockers: propranolol (Inderal), nadolol (Corgard), metoprolol (Lopressor), pindolol (Visken)

TABLE 6-2. POSSIBLE MEDICATION FOR CHILDREN WITH AUTISM SPECTRUM DISORDERS, CONTINUED	
Coexisting Condition	**Medication Considerations**
Sleep disturbances	Melatonin agonists: melatonin,[a] ramelteon (Rozerem)
	Antihistamines: diphenhydramine (Benadryl), hydroxyzine (Atarax, Vistaril)
	Alpha-2 agonists: clonidine (Catapres, Kapvay), guanfacine (Tenex, Intuniv)
	Atypical antidepressants: mirtazapine (Remeron), trazodone (Desyrel)
Anxiety	SSRIs: fluoxetine[a] (Prozac), fluvoxamine[a] (Luvox), citalopram (Celexa), escitalopram (Lexapro), paroxetine (Paxil), sertraline (Zoloft)
	Buspirone (Buspar)
	Mirtazapine (Remeron)
Depression	SSRIs: fluoxetine[a] (Prozac), fluvoxamine[a] (Luvox), citalopram (Celexa), escitalopram (Lexapro), paroxetine (Paxil), sertraline (Zoloft)
	Atypical antidepressants: bupropion (Wellbutrin), mirtazapine (Remeron)
Bipolar disorder	Anticonvulsant mood stabilizers: carbamazepine (Tegretol), gabapentin (Neurontin), lamotrigine (Lamictal), oxcarbazepine (Trileptal), topiramate (Topamax), valproic acid (Depakene, Depakote)
	Atypical antipsychotic agents: risperidone (Risperdal), aripiprazole (Abilify), olanzapine (Zyprexa), quetiapine (Seroquel), ziprasidone (Geodon)
	Lithium

Abbreviation: SSRI, selective serotonin reuptake inhibitor.

[a]At least one published double-blind, placebo-controlled trial supports use in patients with an autism spectrum disorder.

Adapted with permission: Scott M. Myers, MD, Chris Plauché Johnson, MD, MEd, the Council on Children With Disabilities. Management of Children With Autism Spectrum Disorders, *Pediatrics,* Volume 120, Page 1169, Copyright 2007 by the American Academy of Pediatrics.

A Few Precautions

Most of the medicines listed in Table 6-2 have not been directly studied in children with ASDs. Those that have the highest level of evidence to support their use in patients with ASDs have been indicated with a superscript [a].

Selective Serotonin Reuptake Inhibitors

Chances are you've heard about this category of medications, which includes drugs like fluoxetine (Prozac), citalopram (Celexa), and sertraline (Zoloft). These may be prescribed for repetitive behaviors, OCD, anxiety, and depression. Studies show that these medications may help in addressing irritability, tantrums, aggression, and difficulty with transitions. Potential side effects of selective serotonin reuptake inhibitors (SSRIs) include nausea, drowsiness, fatigue, abdominal discomfort, headache, dry mouth, hyperactivity, agitation, and changes in sleep.

Studies of SSRIs have shown a small increase in suicidal thoughts compared with placebo (an inactive substance used instead of medicine), particularly among adolescents and young adults. Data also demonstrate, however, that since SSRIs have been used for treating depression in children and adolescents, teen suicides have steadily decreased. While the safety and benefits of SSRIs far outweigh the infrequent side effects, using the medication warrants close monitoring of your child's response.

Stimulants

While it may seem counterintuitive, some children with hyperactivity, impulsivity, and inattention are prescribed stimulants, including methylphenidate (Ritalin) and dextroamphetamine (Dexedrine). There are many preparations available, varying mainly in the duration of effect. Stimulants are most effective in children who strictly have ADHD and less so in children who have ASDs and symptoms of ADHD. Stimulants also may cause more adverse side effects in children with ASDs. Potential side effects include loss of appetite, insomnia, jitteriness, abdominal discomfort, increased heart rate, and irritability. They can also make tics worse and increase anxiety and repetitive behaviors. Concerns about potential serious cardiac side effects are restricted to adults, children with congenital heart disease, and those with a family history of sudden death.

Alpha-2 Agonists

Alpha-2 agonists are prescribed for high blood pressure, but in children with ASDs, they may be used to control aggression, explosive outbursts, and self-injurious behaviors. They are used to treat hyperactivity, impulsiveness, and inattention. These drugs are also first-line agents for reducing tics. As mentioned earlier in the chapter, they can be used to ease sleep problems as well. Common drugs in this category include clonidine (Catapres, Kapvay) and guanfacine (Tenex, Intuniv). Possible side effects of clonidine and guanfacine include drowsiness, dry mouth, decreased blood pressure, dizziness, constipation, and irritability.

Selective Norepinephrine Reuptake Inhibitors

Atomoxetine (Strattera) is a different, non-stimulant medicine prescribed to reduce ADHD symptoms such as distractibility, hyperactivity, and impulsivity while increasing attention. It may be beneficial for children who are sensitive to the side effects of stimulant medication. Common side effects include fatigue, headache, and stomachache.

Atypical Antipsychotics

Atypical antipsychotics, also known as atypical neuroleptics, are a newer generation of medicines used to treat bipolar disorder, schizophrenia, and pronounced agitation and aggression, as well as tics. This newer class of antipsychotics has fewer side effects than those that were used in the past. These drugs include risperidone (Risperdal) and aripiprazole (Abilify), the only 2 drugs specifically approved by the FDA as of this writing for use in children with ASDs. Side effects include diabetes, weight gain, high cholesterol, sleepiness, headaches, and dizziness. Additional complications of some atypical antipsychotics include possible movement disorders and changes in the way the heart keeps rhythm.

Use Medications With Caution

Using psychopharmacologic medications in children with ASDs is a serious step in managing your child's health. As the parent, you should be told exactly how the medication should benefit your child's behavior, when you may expect to see a difference, the side effects he might experience, and what you will do if the treatment does not work. You should work with your child's pediatrician or mental health practitioner to figure out a way to determine the success or failure of a medication. Evaluating a medication may involve talking to teachers, therapists, and aides who work closely with your child. It's also important to follow up with your child's doctor on a regular basis to figure out if adjustments in the medication are needed and if it is possible to safely go off the medication. If any information is unclear to you, you should persist in asking questions.

Typically, medication is started at low doses and gradually increased as tolerated until you've reached a conclusion about its effectiveness. This is called the trial period. During this time there will be frequent follow-up visits and phone calls to ensure safety and make sure your child is responding appropriately. Once the medicine begins working as desired, ongoing monitoring may be less frequent.

What You Should Know About Medications

Putting any child on medication requires close vigilance but is especially important in children who have ASDs. Even over-the-counter medicines and supplements should be closely monitored. Here are some guidelines you should keep in mind.

- Always give the medication exactly as it is prescribed. Follow the dosage and timing requirements closely, and ask your pediatrician or pharmacist what to do if you forget to give your child the medicine on time.
- Do not stop, restart, increase, or decrease any medicine without discussing it with your child's doctor first. If a medicine stops working, your child may need a different dose or schedule. But never make the change yourself without talking to the pediatrician first.
- Keep all medicines out of your child's reach and stored in childproof bottles. Supervise him whenever he takes his medication. Call your child's pediatrician, the hospital emergency department, or poison control if you suspect he has taken too much of a medicine.

- Always tell your pediatrician about other medications your child is taking before he starts taking a new one. You should also tell the doctor about any vitamins, herbal medicines, or diet supplements. Taking more than one medicine at a time may cause more side effects than from either medicine alone and may also lessen the effect of one or the other.
- Alert your child's doctor if you suspect your child is taking street drugs or alcohol. You should also tell your doctor if you suspect your child is pregnant.
- Use one pharmacy for all of your child's medications. Certain medications can interact with one another and cause reactions ranging from mild to fatal. If your child has more than one doctor prescribing medications, each doctor may not know about other drugs your child is taking. Using one pharmacy will allow the pharmacist to review all the medicines your child is taking.
- Store medications properly. Ask the pharmacist where you should keep medications. Some pills are affected by the humidity in a bathroom, while other liquid drugs require refrigeration.
- Measure your medications carefully. If it's in a liquid form, ask for a syringe or dropper. Do not use tableware.

While medications may help with conditions that are common in children with ASDs, some parents may prefer other types of interventions. The next chapter will address these treatments, more commonly known as complementary and alternative medicine.

CHAPTER 7

The Role of Complementary and Alternative Medicine

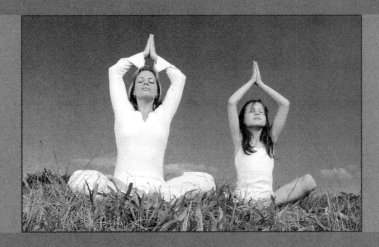

"When my son was diagnosed with autism, my wife and I were like any other parents who'd just been told their child had a lifelong condition: We were prepared to do anything we could to help him reach his full potential. In addition to intensive behavioral therapy, we did a lot of research into nutritional supplements. Although the research showed the supplements were safe, it also said there was limited evidence that they would be helpful in reducing the symptoms of autism. Still, we did try various supplements. After some time, we realized that his progress with behavioral therapy was no better with the supplements than without, so we discontinued them."—Dr Carbone

It's not uncommon for parents of children with special health care needs to turn to complementary and alternative medicine (CAM). In fact, studies show that 30% to 90% of all children with autism spectrum disorders (ASDs) have been put on CAM treatments to address their health problems.

Parents turn to CAM treatments for many reasons. Many parents are afraid of putting their children on conventional medications and worry about the side effects of these treatments. Some have had little success with conventional medications and therapies. Others cannot afford behavioral therapies or do not have easy access to them. Many people believe that CAM treatments are more natural, simpler to use, and less invasive. Some people have benefitted from CAM treatments themselves and want to give their child the same opportunity for benefits. For others, CAM treatments are easier to access.

In this chapter, we'll take a look at some CAM therapies that are often considered for children with ASDs. As any parent who has ever done research on the Internet can tell you, there are hundreds of Web sites that discuss alternative remedies for autism, many with unproven claims. The goal is to help you understand what these treatments are, how they're supposed to benefit children with ASDs, and whether you should consider one of these therapies for your child. We'll also help you evaluate the safety of these treatments and assess whether the benefits are worth the risk.

What Is Complementary and Alternative Medicine (CAM), Exactly?

Complementary and alternative medicine encompasses a host of different therapies. To understand them, it helps to dissect the terminology. *Conventional medicine* (sometimes called Western medicine) refers to treatments that a medical doctor (MD or DO) is likely to prescribe. This is considered "mainstream medicine" and is the most widely used form of medical treatment in the US health care system.

Complementary medicine is a treatment or therapy used in combination with conventional medicine. For example, massage, guided imagery, and acupuncture may be used in addition to analgesic medications to decrease pain.

Alternative medicine is a treatment given in place of a conventional one; for example, some adolescents use herbs rather than antidepressant medication to treat depression.

Taken together, *complementary and alternative medicine,* or CAM, represents a large and diverse group of health care systems, practices, and products that are based on philosophies and techniques other than those used in conventional medicine. Health care professionals who practice *integrative medicine* use a combination of conventional and complementary treatments to treat their patients.

When it comes to treating disease, conventional medicine relies primarily on biomedicine, which is based on the laws of science and the use of the scientific method for evidence. Most treatments are biomedical and based on research, in particular a model known as the randomized, controlled clinical trial (RCT). In an RCT, some subjects are given a treatment and

---

MORE ABOUT INTEGRATIVE MEDICINE

Integrative medicine is primarily relationship-based care. Integrative medicine reaffirms the importance of the relationship between the practitioner and the patient, emphasizes wellness and the inherent drive toward healing, and focuses on the whole person, using all appropriate therapies to achieve the patient's goals for health and healing. It combines mainstream and complementary therapies for which there is some high-quality scientific evidence of safety and effectiveness to promote health for the whole person in the context of the patient's family and community.

others are not, but the researchers do not know who receives the treatment and who doesn't. The research is typically published in a peer-reviewed academic journal. This means it's been closely scrutinized by a panel of medical experts, peers of the researchers who practice in the field that is being studied. The peer-review process is designed to maintain professional, ethical, and scientific standards and provide credibility to the study. In addition, peer review determines if an academic study is suitable for publication in a peer-reviewed journal or other publication.

Many alternative remedies have not undergone such rigorous scrutiny. Instead, support for these treatments is often anecdotal, meaning it's based on casual observations or a story about a person or a situation. This evidence is not as reliable as that from an RCT. All cases or anecdotes are not represented, and anecdotal data are difficult to verify as being an accurate representation of the situation. Sometimes an individual response is inappropriately generalized for all people. The scientific method cannot be used in most cases to investigate anecdotal data. The scientific method uses careful written observation and collection of measurable data to answer questions through carefully designed experiments. Anecdotal data can become a testimonial to help promote a product or an idea.

Just because an alternative treatment has not been subjected to an RCT does not mean it will not work. It's possible, too, that some alternative remedies may benefit from the placebo effect, in which the patient's faith in the treatment—or the practitioner delivering it—may be enough to bring about a positive effect.

For any parent considering a CAM treatment for a child with an ASD, the most important thing you can do is to become educated and use common sense. Know the potential benefits of the treatments and understand the risks involved. Your pediatrician can help you in this process, and together you can decide whether or not to pursue the treatment. (See Figure 7-1.) It's also important to know the resources needed to start and maintain the therapy. Many of these therapies can be quite costly. It is important for parents to investigate if a CAM therapy has been researched in an evidence-based scientific study. You can often find these studies on university or national accredited Web sites such as the National Institutes of Health (www.ncbi.nlm.nih.gov/pubmed).

FIGURE 7-1. A COMMONSENSE GUIDE TO COMPLEMENTARY AND ALTERNATIVE MEDICINE TREATMENT RECOMMENDATIONS			
		Is the therapy effective?	
		Yes	*No*
Is the therapy safe?	*Yes*	Recommend	Tolerate
	No	Monitor closely or discourage	Discourage

From Kemper K, Cohen M. Ethics meet complementary and alternative medicine: new light on old principles. *Contemp Pediatr.* 2004;21:65

Gluten-free/Casein-free Diet

Back in the 1960s, a physician named F. Curtis Dohan speculated that people who had celiac disease were more likely to have schizophrenia. Celiac disease is an autoimmune disorder in which the body cannot tolerate gluten, a protein found naturally in wheat, as well as rye, barley, and sometimes oats that are processed in the same place as these other grains. Later studies have not established that reducing the amount of wheat in the diet of people with schizophrenia significantly reduces their symptoms. Dohan's writings marked the beginning of the proposed link between diet and psychiatric and neurologic illnesses.

The suggested link between gluten and casein and autism emerged in the 1970s. The theory—which remains unproven—was that children who have ASDs are unable to break down the dietary proteins in gluten and casein, causing the formation of opioid-like peptides (amino acids that are similar to proteins). Children with autism are also believed to have "leaky gut syndrome." Because of this syndrome, these peptides are then able to escape from the digestive tract, cross the intestinal membranes, enter the bloodstream, and go up to the brain, causing the neurobehavioral symptoms that we know as ASDs. By eliminating foods that contain gluten and casein from a child's diet (known as the gluten-free/casein-free [GFCF] diet), it was believed that you could diminish the symptoms of autism.

Some parents say that the GFCF diet has lessened their child's symptoms. Research, however, has found little support for the GFCF diet and "leaky gut" theory. Several studies of the GFCF diet in children with ASDs have shown that removing gluten and casein from a child's diet did not improve social skills or communication, nor did it help with sleep duration and activity levels. Even so, it's possible that some children with ASDs who have significant gastrointestinal problems may reap some benefits from the GFCF diet, especially if they, coincidentally, also have celiac disease (gluten-sensitivity autoimmune disorder).

Still, many parents try removing gluten and casein from their child's diet. In fact, the GFCF diet is the most popular CAM intervention among children who have ASDs. It's generally considered safe, and some parents report that the diet has actually made a difference in their child's behavior. But it's hard to know if these behavioral changes are directly related to the GFCF diet or if they are the result of another intervention that the child may be undergoing at the same time.

It's possible, too, that some children are lactose intolerant, meaning they can't tolerate the sugar in milk, which may cause gastrointestinal distress leading to irritability. Others may actually have celiac disease, which can also cause behavioral disturbances. By removing lactose and gluten in children who have these conditions, you may also notice behavioral improvements.

Should You Try It?

While the available science does not support the GFCF diet, it is understandable that some parents will want to try this intervention. After all, it's something that you can control and do on your own, and it is thought to be relatively safe. Before you do anything, though, talk with your child's pediatrician first. You may also want to speak with a nutritionist because the GFCF diet may place your child at risk for some nutritional deficiencies.

For example, eliminating all milk products from your child's diet removes a critical source of calcium and vitamin D, key nutrients essential for strong bones. New evidence suggests that vitamin D may also play a role in the immune system and preventing infections, cancer, and diabetes. In addition, your child may require additional sources of protein because dairy products are often a major source of protein in a child's diet. Of note, however, is that these needed minerals are not always included in the now-popular "gummy" type vitamins.

Taking gluten out of your child's diet can pose challenges too. Removing grains like wheat, barley, rye, and oats from your child's diet eliminates important nutrients such as the B vitamins, iron, and fiber. Children who do the GFCF diet may benefit from vitamin and mineral supplements to make up for the nutrients missing from their daily diet.

Doing the diet can be difficult too. Gluten isn't always easy to detect, and reading labels can be challenging. While some sources like bread, pasta, and cereal may be obvious, others such as deli meats, salad dressings, and broths may be less so. And if your child is already a picky eater, it may be a challenge to convince him to adopt this new way of eating. Food preparation may be more time-consuming for children on a GFCF diet, and the cost of the diet can be higher than a traditional diet for children.

ALTERNATIVE SOURCES OF KEY NUTRIENTS

If you decide to put your child on the gluten-free/casein-free diet, it's important to pay attention to certain nutrients such as vitamin D, calcium, iron, protein, and fiber, which may be lacking in this eating plan. The following chart offers other options for getting these important nutrients:

NUTRIENT NEEDS	ALTERNATIVE SOURCES
Vitamin D	Fortified rice, soy, and almond milk; cod liver oil; tofu, eggs; short-term exposure to sunlight; supplements
Calcium	Fortified rice, soy, and almond milk; fortified orange juice; beans, broccoli, spinach, kale, tofu, tempeh; supplements
Iron	Red meats, pork, chicken (mainly in dark meat), shellfish, egg yolks, spinach, soybean nuts, prunes, raisins; supplements
Protein	Eggs, nuts and seeds, lean meats, beans, peanut butter
Fiber	Legumes, fruits, vegetables, nuts, seeds; supplements

While the GFCF diet is certainly among the most popular eating plans used in children with ASDs, you may also hear about diets that restrict certain foods or nutrients. Before putting your child on any type of diet, talk with your child's pediatrician first. You'll need to make sure your child is receiving all the nutrients important for his growth and development.

Dietary Supplements

The number of children and adults taking nutritional supplements has grown significantly in recent years. Multivitamins are the most common CAM treatment—as many as 41% of children take a daily multivitamin. Among teenagers, as many as 75% take herbal remedies and other dietary supplements. It is not surprising that parents of children with ASDs are interested in these same treatments to support the health of their children.

Vitamin B$_6$ and Magnesium

Vitamin B$_6$, or pyridoxine, helps the body make serotonin and norepinephrine, 2 important chemical messengers in the brain. Vitamin B$_6$ also helps produce enzymes for metabolizing protein and red blood cells. Children who do not get enough vitamin B$_6$ are at risk for certain skin conditions, nerve problems, irritability, and depression.

Magnesium is an essential mineral that is involved in more than 300 biochemical reactions in the body. It's required for proper brain and muscle function, metabolism, and bone and immune health. Magnesium helps to convert the amino acid 5-hydroxytryptophan into serotonin, a chemical messenger involved in regulating mood and keeping depression and anxiety at bay.

Back in the 1960s, some experts began to suggest that certain forms of mental illness were linked to biochemical problems in the body and that using vitamins as therapy could correct them. In children with ASDs, some people thought that the body was unable to convert vitamin B$_6$ into a compound required to produce dopamine, a chemical messenger in the brain that regulates movement and behavior. Many children with ASDs were also believed to have low levels of magnesium, though there was no direct connection to autism.

Giving children a high-dose combination of vitamin B_6 and magnesium is a common CAM treatment for children with ASDs but is based largely on observations, not strong science. Some studies using low doses showed no benefits. Other studies using higher doses suggested that there might be some improvement in language or attention, but the research was not well designed.

Always talk with your child's pediatrician before you attempt this kind of a therapy. Treatment has potentially dangerous side effects, including peripheral neuropathy (nerve damage that can cause numbness, pain, and burning) from too much vitamin B_6, or diarrhea and arrhythmia (an abnormal heart rhythm) from high doses of magnesium.

Omega-3 Fatty Acids

Omega-3 fatty acids, especially docosahexaenoic acid (DHA) and eicosapentaenoic acid (EPA), are essential for healthy brain development and proper communication between brain cells. They occur naturally in fatty fish and certain plant foods. In recent years, these healthy fats have been widely touted for their effects in preventing heart disease and depression. Some studies have suggested that these essential fatty acids might help improve attention, focus, and activity in children who have attention-deficit/hyperactivity disorder (ADHD). Some people believe they may also have a beneficial effect on children with ASDs, although it is not well understood why this would be.

Small-scale research studies have suggested that high doses of omega-3 fatty acids might help in reducing repetitive behaviors such as pacing or rocking, fixated interests, irritability, and hyperactivity in children with ASDs. Evidence, however, is sparse. There is a need for larger scale research studies to better understand the possible benefit of omega-3 fatty acids for children with ASDs.

If you want to give your child omega-3 fatty acid supplements, make sure to talk with your child's pediatrician first. Keep in mind, too, that these fatty acids may cause gastrointestinal problems such as diarrhea, bloating, and abdominal pain. Make sure to identify certain behaviors and keep track of how those behaviors change, so you'll know if the supplements are making a difference. (See Appendix D for sample Medication Flow Sheet.)

Probiotics

The intestines harbor a rich array of bacteria that are responsible for the healthy functioning of our digestive, immune, and nervous systems. Among them are probiotics, nontoxic bacteria or beneficial yeasts that dwell in our gut and are found in certain fermented foods like kefir, yogurt, and tempeh. Probiotics are also available in supplement form as liquids, powders, or capsules. Among the most popular forms are lactobacillus, bifidobacterium, and saccharomyces.

Studies show that about 25% of all children with ASDs take probiotics not for the core symptoms of ASD but for the gastrointestinal and allergy issues that many children, including those with ASDs, face such as diarrhea, constipation, irritable bowel syndrome, eczema, or certain allergies.

A recent review of children who used probiotics found that the probiotics can help reduce the length of viral diarrheal illness and prevent or reduce the severity of antibiotic-associated diarrhea. In certain premature babies, probiotics may protect against a severe gastrointestinal complication known as necrotizing enterocolitis, but more studies are needed. More research also is needed before probiotics can be recommended to treat disorders such as irritable bowel syndrome, Crohn disease, colic, and constipation, and to prevent common infections and allergy in children.

Probiotics are generally considered safe, but in rare cases they may be unsafe in children who are severely debilitated or immune compromised or who live in households where such issues exist.

Multivitamins

As mentioned, multivitamins are the most common CAM treatment. Vitamins are chemicals that the body needs, in small amounts, for many important functions. There are many diseases that result in not having enough of a certain vitamin; in these cases, using a vitamin supplement can be beneficial. In the case of ASD, there are some who suggest that very high doses of certain vitamins are needed. Currently, however, there are no high-quality scientific studies that show that high-dose (above the recommended amount) vitamin therapy is beneficial for children with ASDs. If you suspect that your child may be deficient in certain vitamins or minerals, speak to your child's pediatrician. Various studies have shown that children with ASDs may be at risk for nutritional deficiencies as the result of dietary restrictions or from being extremely selective eaters.

In general, vitamins that are given in recommended amounts are safe. The problem is that sometimes children wind up taking too much of certain vitamins, which causes toxicity. If you decide to give your child multivitamins and supplements, it's important to read labels and not give your child too much of any individual vitamin, especially the fat-soluble vitamins A, D, E, and K. Know the tolerable upper intake levels for individual vitamins in healthy children, and make sure your child's daily intake doesn't exceed these levels (see "Beware of Too Much" on the next page).

Vitamin C

Vitamin C is a water-soluble vitamin responsible for healing, immune function, and iron absorption. It plays a key role in producing the neurotransmitters (chemical signals in the brain) norepinephrine and serotonin and in the breakdown of dopamine, another chemical messenger. These neurotransmitters play important roles in regulating mood, attention, and coordination and managing stress.

One small-scale study found that vitamin C in children with ASDs reduced stereotypic behaviors, but there are no well-designed studies of the effects of vitamin C supplements in children with ASDs. Vitamin C is rarely used as a sole treatment for autism, but it may be part of a regimen of supplements, especially if there are concerns about vitamin C deficiency. It is a relatively safe supplement, though high doses may cause gastrointestinal problems such as diarrhea and kidney stones.

BEWARE OF TOO MUCH			

Some vitamins can be dangerous at high levels. Here's what experts recommend daily as well as daily upper limits.

VITAMIN	AGE	DAILY RECOMMENDED INTAKE	DAILY TOLERABLE UPPER INTAKE LEVEL
Vitamin A	Infants 0–6 months	400 µg/1,320 IU	600 µg/1,980 IU
	Infants 7–12 months	500 µg/1,650 IU	600 µg/1,980 IU
	Children 1–3 years	300 µg/990 IU	600 µg/1,980 IU
	Children 4–8 years	400 µg/1,320 IU	900 µg/2,970 IU
	Children 9–13 years	600 µg/1,980 IU	1,700 µg/5,610 IU
	Girls 14–18 years	700 µg/2,310 IU	2,800 µg/9,240 IU
	Boys 14–18 years	900 µg/2,970 IU	2,800 µg/9,240 IU
Vitamin D	Infants 0–12 months	5 µg/200 IU	25 µg/1,000 IU
	Children 1–18 years	5 µg/200 IU	50 µg/2,000 IU
Vitamin E	Infants 0–6 months	4 mg/9.3 µmol	Not determinable
	Infants 7–12 months	5 mg/11.6 µmol	Not determinable
	Children 1–3 years	6 mg/13.9 µmol	200 mg/464 µmol
	Children 4–8 years	7 mg/16.3 µmol	300 mg/696 µmol
	Children 9–13 years	11 mg/25.6 µmol	600 mg/1,392 µmol
	Children 14–18 years	15 mg/34.9 µmol	800 mg/1,856 µmol

Source: This table was created based on content from the American Academy of Pediatrics *Pediatric Nutrition Handbook,* 6th Edition, 2009, and updated as of June 2011.

Melatonin

Many children with ASDs have trouble getting a good night's sleep. For those who have trouble falling asleep, melatonin may be a good option. Melatonin is a hormone naturally secreted by the pineal gland in the brain that helps to regulate our body's sleep-wake cycles. Some studies have found that children with ASDs have low melatonin levels.

Melatonin has been found through RCTs to be safe and effective at reducing the amount of time it takes for children who have difficulties falling asleep to doze off and increasing the length of time spent sleeping. (It is not generally used, though, to *keep* a child asleep.) Better sleep in these children (and their caregivers!) may lead to better daytime behavior and less family stress. Potential side effects of melatonin include nightmares and nighttime waking. If your child is having difficulty falling or staying asleep, your pediatrician can help you decide if melatonin might be helpful.

A PARENT'S STORY: RONNY

"Bedtime was always a struggle for us. Our son CJ, who is now 4, would scream for 2 hours straight. So my partner and I would split up and each take 1 child. By the time he was done screaming and crying, the parent with CJ would wind up asleep in his room. Once, he climbed out and crawled into his brother's crib.

"Our doctor suggested melatonin. Every night he gets a cup of milk with melatonin dissolved in it. Then we do his nightly routine. He brushes his teeth, reads a book and says, 'Daddy, it's time for bed.' Melatonin has been a lifesaver."

Supplements for Oxidative Stress

Some researchers believe that oxidative stress and toxicity—when our bodies produce and cannot get rid of toxic forms of oxygen—are the culprits behind the neuronal (nerve cell) problems in children with ASDs. Certain supplements are believed to help rid the body of this oxidative stress and enhance immune function. These include

- *Dimethylglycine.* Dimethylglycine is a by-product of the amino acid glycine. It is found naturally in some foods, like beans and liver, and is available as a supplement. Some early reports suggested that dimethylglycine might improve speech and behavior in people who have ASDs, but more studies are needed. This supplement is generally considered safe but may cause hyperactivity as a side effect.
- *Methylcobalamin.* Also known as methyl B_{12}, this supplement is involved in the proper functioning of certain antioxidants such as glutathione and a chemical process in the body called methylation. Some people believe that autism is the result of faulty methylation, which results in the expression of genes that cause ASDs. Methylation is also important for ridding the body of oxidative stress. There have been no well-designed, controlled studies of the effect of methyl B_{12} supplements on the behavior of children with ASDs.
- *Folic acid, folinic acid, and folate.* These are all forms of a water-soluble B vitamin and are best known for preventing neural tube defects in unborn babies. Folate is sometimes given in conjunction with methyl B_{12} to increase levels of glutathione. They are also believed to increase levels of S-adenosylhomocysteine, or SAM-e, which is important for the production, activation, and breakdown of several important chemical messengers in the brain. There have been no well-designed studies of the effect of folate, folic acid, or folinic acid supplements, with or without methyl B_{12}, on the behavior of children with ASDs.

Amino Acids

Amino acids play a critical role in the brain. In fact, many neurotransmitters are amino acids themselves or derived from amino acids. Not surprisingly, amino acids are essential for mental health and well-being.

Two amino acids that have been used in children with ASDs are carnosine and carnitine. Carnosine has antioxidant properties and is believed to benefit brain health. Carnitine is found primarily in meat and is responsible for cellular energy production. There are not enough high-quality studies to say that carnosine or carnitine supplements are helpful for children with ASDs. So while both amino acids are generally considered safe and well-tolerated, there is little science showing that they have any efficacy in autism.

Interventions That Eliminate Infections

Through the years, there has been no shortage of theories about what causes autism. A weakened immune system that falls prey to viruses, bacteria, and fungi has been suggested as a possible cause of ASDs. Although the immune system may be affected in some children with ASDs, there is no strong scientific evidence supporting the theory that problems with the immune system cause autism.

Intravenous Immunoglobulin

Research in recent years has found that some children who have ASDs have different immune systems compared with their typical peers. For instance, research has found irregular levels of cytokines, substances that regulate important bodily immune functions. As a result, some people believe that altering the immune system may affect symptoms of ASDs and have tried giving their children oral or intravenous immunoglobulin (IVIG) treatment. Intravenous immunoglobulin, which comes from human plasma, is used to treat neurologic diseases rooted in autoimmune problems such as myasthenia gravis and Guillain-Barré syndrome. Unfortunately, studies have generally shown that IVIG does not help to decrease or eliminate symptoms of ASDs. The treatment is also costly and may cause serious side effects, including infection from contaminated blood products (such as viral hepatitis or HIV), meningitis, anaphylactic shock, kidney failure, decreased urination, sudden weight gain, swelling of the legs or ankles, or shortness of breath.

Antiviral Agents

Although no specific virus has been identified as the cause of autism, some people believe that treating children with antiviral agents can help. The theory behind these medications is that autism is the result of a chronic viral infection of the central nervous system. There are no clinical trials at all that show antiviral agents are helpful in reducing or eliminating symptoms of ASDs. In fact, overusing these agents may be dangerous and risks suppressing bone marrow, the thick inner part of bone that produces white blood cells, red blood cells, and platelets. Other side effects include nausea, dizziness, headache, abdominal pain, and depression.

Antibiotics

Looking back, many parents recall their child suffering several ear infections before being diagnosed with an ASD. These infections were most often treated with antibiotics that some people believe may have altered gut microflora. These microflora are believed by some to promote the growth of bacteria that harm the nervous system, which in turn contributes to the development of autism.

Certain antibiotics have been used to try and clear the gut of the presumed toxic bacteria, but there is currently no research showing that antibiotics can help reduce symptoms of ASDs. Using antibiotics for a prolonged time is discouraged because it can lead to antibiotic resistance and can cause colitis, a sometimes serious inflammation of the colon.

Anti-yeast Treatments

Although there is no evidence to support this theory, some believe that overgrowth of a particular yeast, *Candida,* in the intestines may play some role in the development of autism. It is believed that the excess yeast, in turn, causes the symptoms we know as autism. To tame *Candida* overgrowth, some people give their children antifungal medications, which may cause harmful side effects. Chronic use of fluconazole, a prescription antifungal agent, may result in liver toxicity and an itchy skin condition known as exfoliative dermatitis. Nystatin, another antifungal agent, may cause diarrhea. Furthermore, no clinical trials have been done to evaluate antifungal effectiveness in reducing ASD symptoms.

Nonbiological Interventions

Changing behavior is also possible with nonbiological therapies. Some of these may even alter the underlying neural makeup in the brain. Among those used in ASDs include the following:

Auditory Integration Therapy

Auditory integration therapy is an intervention that conditions children with ASDs to tolerate certain sounds by listening to filtered music in a sound booth over a period of time. It is designed to retrain the ear to process sounds in a more normal fashion without any distortions. The cost of these sessions however, can be quite expensive, and the evidence to date does not support its use in treating ASDs.

Sensory Integration Therapy

Sensory integration therapy is a form of occupational therapy that you may recall reading about in Chapter 4. The therapist may place the child in a specially designed room that stimulates all of her senses. During a typical session, the therapist works with the child to encourage movement and elicit appropriate responses to various sensory stimuli. Therapy is based on the assumption that the child is overstimulated or under-stimulated by her environment and that therapy can improve her ability to process sensory input.

Despite dozens of studies over the past 4 decades, research about the effectiveness of sensory integration therapy is still insufficient to move this popular intervention into the realm of standard therapies for ASDs.

Behavioral Optometry

The chance that a child with an ASD will have a vision problem is thought to be no different than in a child with typical development. Currently there is inadequate evidence to suggest that eye or vision problems cause or increase symptoms of ASDs. Some professionals, however, believe that certain vision therapies might benefit a child's behavior—especially those associated with learning disabilities, language disorders, and other developmental problems—by improving his visual functioning. It is based on the belief that the problem behavior is actually the result of faulty eye movement.

Behavioral optometry is generally not recommended in children with ASDs or those who have learning disabilities. In fact, in 2011, the American Academy of Pediatrics (AAP), along with the American Association for Pediatric Ophthalmology and Strabismus and the American Academy of Ophthalmology, issued a joint technical report saying that "Scientific evidence does not support the claims that visual training, muscle exercises, ocular pursuit-and-tracking exercises, behavioral/perceptual vision therapy, 'training' glasses, prisms, and colored lenses and filters are effective direct or indirect treatments for learning disabilities."

Craniosacral Therapy

Craniosacral therapy involves applying pressure to manipulate the fluid around the brain. The practice is usually performed by a chiropractor or motor therapist. The gentle pressure is intended to improve the function of the central nervous system and relieve stress. Research,

---

A PARENT'S STORY: CARLY

"Our son Asher, who is now 7, suffers from a great deal of anxiety. For him, deep pressure on his body has always worked best at relaxing him. These days, he likes to put his head into my neck and just nestle against me. Then he wants me to wrap my arms around him and just squeeze.

"Not surprisingly, Asher always responded best to forms of massage, in particular therapeutic brushing and joint compression. Therapeutic brushing involves brushing a small surgical brush on his arms and legs in soft, rhythmic strokes. I follow that with joint compression, in which I gently pressed together the joints at his shoulder, elbow, knees, and ankles for quick counts of 10. For some reason, when I did those 2 things every 2 hours, it would make my son more focused. It's as if it triggered something in his brain that helped him form his mouth better to make sounds. Unfortunately, he grew immune to its effects after 6 months.

"I also used to lie [down] on his back or roll a yoga ball from his back down to his feet. The weight of my body and the yoga ball soothed him and reduced his anxiety. But he doesn't like those techniques anymore. He still wears a weighted blanket at times, which helps reduce his stress, but I don't think it's heavy enough. He has found that he enjoys the deep pressure much more in an upright position.

"We did try him on the GFCF diet for a while when he was 4, but it was hard because he saw his sisters and parents eating the foods he really wanted, which made him upset. Also, during those 3 weeks, Asher was very lethargic and solemn. My happy little boy who once had lots of energy and loved to play all of a sudden wasn't happy anymore. His teachers would tell me that he didn't want to play or participate and just wanted to sit in a corner alone. It was an awful experience. We discontinued it after 3 weeks.

"Now, we use melatonin every night. He takes [it] before bedtime. He winds up very tired, sleeps well, and wakes up refreshed. That has worked very well."

Carly's story illustrates how families are the experts in caring for their children and in determining how some of the complementary and alternative medicine therapies discussed in this chapter are beneficial for their children. As you consider various therapies, be sure to discuss all options with your child's pediatrician.

however, has found that simply touching the area around the spine does not alter the pressure of cerebrospinal fluid. Craniosacral therapy is not recommended in children who have Down syndrome because of possible neck bone problems that risk injury to the spinal cord. Although massage can be an effective way to relax a child who has an ASD, there is no evidence that craniosacral therapy has any benefit on core symptoms of ASDs.

CAM Therapies to Avoid

Over the years, parents of children with ASDs have turned to numerous therapies with the hope of helping their children. Some of these treatments have turned out to be harmful and potentially deadly.

Chelation

For years, many people believed—and some still do—that autism was caused by thimerosal, a preservative used in vaccines that contains mercury. This alleged link has been scientifically disproved in numerous studies and reports. Still, the notion spawned interest in a treatment called chelation, a treatment that binds to heavy metals in the body and allows them to be excreted in the urine. Chelation also binds to other metals in the body, including iron and calcium, which are important and essential nutrients. Chelation is approved by the US Food and Drug Administration for treating lead poisoning but is not approved for autism.

Several chelating agents are available, and some are sold over the counter. Two of the most common are ethylenediaminetetraacetic acid (EDTA) and meso-2,3-dimercaptosuccinic acid (DMSA). Treatment may be given orally or intravenously, or applied topically to the skin.

Because chelation is a potentially dangerous treatment, it should not be used to treat ASDs. Using chelation intravenously is especially dangerous and has resulted in the death of a child. It has not been studied in people with ASDs, and any reports of its effectiveness have been subjective.

Hyperbaric Oxygen Therapy

Hyperbaric oxygen therapy (HBOT) involves placing the patient in a large, non-portable container, and increasing air pressure to levels just slightly higher than normal atmospheric levels and boosting oxygen levels to 100%. It's generally used to treat a condition in scuba divers known as "the bends," which occurs when they surface too quickly and develop oxygen bubbles in their blood. It's also used to treat carbon monoxide poisoning and burns. As a treatment for autism, HBOT is intended to correct the theorized abnormal oxygen metabolism in the brains of children with ASDs and eliminate excess oxygen.

Most studies have found that HBOT is ineffective in treating autism, and the treatment is potentially dangerous. Side effects include ear pain, reversible nearsightedness, and seizures. Because of the potential for harm and lack of good scientific evidence of its benefit, HBOT is not recommended to treat autism.

Secretin

Using secretin to treat autism has largely disappeared, but it enjoyed a great deal of popularity in the late 1990s. Secretin is an intestinal hormone that controls digestion. In 1998, an uncontrolled study (there was no control group to compare against subjects who received treatment) involving just 3 children showed that secretin relieved some of the communication and social skill deficits of autism while also helping with gastrointestinal symptoms. Excitement soon died down, however, when more than 15 controlled studies consistently showed clear evidence that secretin lacked benefit. Today it is no longer regarded as a treatment for autism.

TESTS YOUR CHILD DOESN'T NEED

In recent years, some parents have been urged to get tests on their children that are entirely unnecessary in diagnosing autism spectrum disorders. These tests include hair analysis, micronutrient levels (such as vitamin levels), intestinal permeability studies, stool analysis, urinary peptides, and mercury level. These tests are not needed and are quite expensive to obtain.

Mind-Body Therapies

Children with ASDs who are high functioning and have good language skills may benefit from some CAM therapies that help a child regulate emotions and maintain a state of calm. Although these treatments do not yet have the science behind them, they do offer an alternative to psychotropic medications, which may cause unpleasant side effects and are often expensive. Among them are

- *Yoga.* This ancient physical and spiritual discipline and philosophy originated in India more than 5,000 years ago. Today, it's a popular form of exercise that uses poses or postures to strengthen and condition the body while calming and nourishing the mind. The practice is believed to improve concentration, discipline, and confidence while also enhancing flexibility, strength, and coordination. Yoga is already gaining popularity as a treatment for children with ADHD, a condition that often exists in children with ASDs too. It is also showing promise as a treatment for many other ailments such as arthritis, back pain, and insomnia. There are currently no well-designed studies of yoga's effects on symptoms of ASDs, but it has been shown to be a safe activity for children with certain disabilities.

- *Neurofeedback.* Like any form of biofeedback, neurofeedback therapy (NFT) "feeds back" information about a patient's physiologic functioning. In NFT the patient learns to regulate or control physiologic impulses in the brain and then change outward behaviors. Studies about whether or not NFT is effective are not conclusive. In some children with ASDs, neurofeedback has reportedly improved behavior and reduced symptoms. The National Institute of Mental Health is now funding a trial on NFT for children with ASDs; at this time, however, there is no evidence that NFT improves symptoms of ASDs. On the other hand, initial studies examining NFT for symptoms of ADHD suggest that there may be an improvement in brain function in that disorder. It may be that children with ASDs who seem to benefit from NFT might be having improvement in coexisting ADHD symptoms rather than a true improvement in the core symptoms of ASDs. This therapy has no side effects but is costly. The scientific evidence does not recommend its use for children with ASDs at this time.

- *Music therapy.* Some people with ASDs display remarkable talent for music, so it's not surprising that therapists have tried to use music to help children with ASDs gain new skills in communication and expression. While there have been some small studies that show encouraging results, more studies are needed to know if music therapy is beneficial for children with ASDs.

Finding a CAM Practitioner

Locating a therapist who practices a CAM treatment isn't as difficult as it once was because these treatments have become increasingly common. For instance, many pediatricians are becoming more knowledgeable about complementary and alternative therapies and can provide advice on these treatments. In fact, the AAP has about 200 pediatricians who are members of its Section on Complementary and Integrative Medicine.

If you are interested in seeking a CAM practitioner, start by talking to your child's pediatrician. Your pediatrician can tell you whether or not a treatment is safe and may also be able to refer you to a licensed practitioner or therapist in your area. Don't be afraid to ask a potential practitioner about credentials, education, and experience. Ask whether the practitioner has experience treating children, in particular those with ASDs. Find out how many children the practitioner has treated and how often they are treated now. Make sure to gather information about office hours, costs, and insurance coverage.

Also, check into your state's licensing requirements for different types of CAM. Some states will require a license to practice acupuncture, for instance, but others do not. In states that do not, check to see if your acupuncturist has been certified by a national professional organization. In fact, it can be quite useful to check if any practitioner, such as an occupational therapist, has additional certification in a particular CAM treatment (such as sensory integration therapy).

If you decide on a CAM treatment, make sure to let your child's pediatrician know. Tell the doctor about any vitamins, supplements, or herbs you give your child. This information is critical because combining these products with a prescribed medication can sometimes produce dangerous side effects. Also, do not stop any prescribed medications without first speaking with your doctor.

Is CAM Covered?

Getting a CAM treatment can be expensive, especially if the therapy isn't covered by your health insurance plan. Some insurance companies are now picking up the tab for these treatments, but coverage depends on the insurance plan you have. Other therapies may be managed and offered by school districts. In some states, families may be able to receive financial assistance from developmental disability agencies. On the other hand, some treatments may not ever be covered, which means you'll have to pay for the entire treatment out of your own pocket. Before seeking a CAM treatment, check with your insurance company to see if it is covered. Ask practitioners what they charge and to specify exactly what will be done.

TOO GOOD TO BE TRUE

Many complementary and alternative therapies lack scientific proof that support their use as autism spectrum disorder treatments and the many health conditions associated with it. Knowing how to spot a false claim is important to avoid being overly persuaded by a treatment with no evidence behind it. Here are 6 kinds of claims to avoid.

- Those that are based on overly simple scientific theories. Your child's pediatrician can help you look into the science behind a therapy.

- Claims that a therapy can treat multiple different, unrelated symptoms, diseases, or conditions.

- Claims that use case reports or subjective data rather than carefully designed studies to show their effectiveness.

- Claims that children will respond dramatically or even experience a cure.

- Claims that say there's no need for controlled studies or peer-reviewed references.

- Claims that the treatment has no potential or reported adverse effects.

Final Word on CAM

It's not unusual for parents of children with ASDs to explore complementary and alternative remedies for their children. Some of these treatments may even offer some benefit. Others, however, may not. Research on these remedies is sparse, and much of the evidence is subjective. But just because something doesn't have scientific evidence backing it up doesn't mean it doesn't work; it simply means that scientists haven't subjected the treatment to rigorous scientific study. Many treatments once considered complementary are now mainstream. As stated earlier, the most important thing you can do is to become educated and use common sense. Know the potential benefits of the treatments and how to measure those effects (see Figure 7-1).

The bottom line is this: if you decide to look into a CAM treatment for your child, do your research. Start by asking your child's pediatrician what she knows about it and whether she can help you understand the potential benefits and risks. Read articles about the treatment on reputable Web sites such as those of the US National Institutes of Health National Center for Complementary and Alternative Medicine, the Consortium of Academic Health Centers for Integrative Medicine, and the Association for Science in Autism Treatment. (See Appendix A for more information.) Find out what the benefits, risks, and potential side effects are of any treatment. And tell your child's pediatrician and other health care practitioners if you decide to use a CAM treatment with your child. Being open and honest about your child's care, as you'll learn in Chapter 8, is the best thing you can do to ensure her health and safety.

Partnering With Your Pediatrician

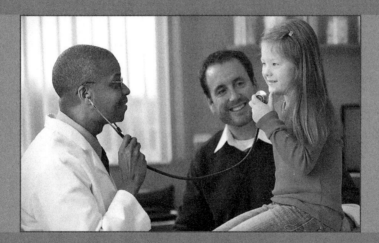

Ideally your child's pediatrician has played a vital role in caring for your child with an autism spectrum disorder (ASD). Your pediatrician may have been the one who listened to you when you had concerns about your child's behavior and development. He may have been the one to screen your child for ASDs, refer you to a specialist or an early intervention (EI) program, and provide you with information and community resources on autism.

There are things you should be able to expect from your pediatrician, but the relationship with your pediatrician is a partnership, one that requires input from you, the parent, not just your doctor. We'll discuss how you can work with your child's pediatrician so that your child receives the best care possible. Good care also involves input from pediatric staff (including nurses, nurse practitioners, and physician assistants), therapists who your child sees, and other medical and educational specialists involved in your child's care. A medical home will help you bring together all the components of your child's care. In this chapter, we'll discuss the medical home concept and why it's so essential to the care and well-being of children with ASDs.

Every child, every patient, is entitled to quality medical care, but it's especially important for children with special health care needs, such as those with ASDs. Children with ASDs tend to have more frequent contact with the health care system. Often, treating children with ASDs demands more of the pediatrician. It may require more time during an office visit to address the needs of the child with an ASD and her family. Many of these children also have other medical conditions.

While some physicians have limited experience with children with ASDs, many pediatricians are now seeing numerous children with ASDs in their practice. In a 2009 survey, doctors reported having about 40 visits with families of children with autism per year. With current rates, each pediatrician will care for about 15 patients with an ASD. Knowing what you can expect from your pediatrician and fulfilling your own responsibilities in this partnership will help ensure that your child gets the care he deserves.

What Should You Expect From Your Pediatrician?

Pediatricians are important advocates for any child but especially for children with special health care needs like ASDs. Here are some key things your pediatrician may do for you if you suspect or know your child has an ASD.

- Listen to all your concerns about your child's development, be it speech and language delays, delays in social skills, or the presence of unusual behaviors. Research has shown that most parents are usually correct when they suspect something is wrong with their child's growth and development.
- Give you a screening questionnaire that will probe more deeply into your child's development.
- Give you a screening questionnaire specific for ASD.
- Refer to a professional or team of professionals who use the latest diagnostic tools to help make a formal diagnosis.
- Refer for an audiology evaluation.
- Refer for EI services in your community even before there is a formal diagnosis.
- Persist in addressing your concerns even if a screening test result is negative.
- Pay close attention to and screen younger siblings of your child with an ASD, given the increased rate of recurrence within families (see Chapter 2).
- Stay abreast of the most recent research and developments in the field of autism and be aware of local agencies, services, and support groups available to you and your children.
- Continue to follow up on the care of your child after the diagnosis, and be an active partner with you in your child's medical home.

You need to be certain that you feel that you can talk to your pediatrician, and that he is able to do these key things. But it takes more than just your pediatrician; children with ASDs need medical homes.

> ### My son's pediatrician knows a lot about autism, but it's difficult to talk with her. How do we deal with this?
>
> When it comes to a condition like autism, a doctor who has the clinical skills, knowledge, and expertise in treating autism spectrum disorders is a definite plus. A doctor is also better able to treat your child's health concerns if she has an interest in that area of medicine. Her experience will ultimately help her direct you to resources and other experts in the community.
>
> But if it is hard to speak with her or if you receive information that is hard to understand, ask that things be described in simpler terms. Or perhaps you can call later to go over your questions. Write a note or tell your pediatrician in person when you are not pleased. Be as specific as possible so it can improve your child's care as well as that of other children. It may help to schedule an extended parent conference with your pediatrician to discuss issues in greater detail than is typically possible at a sick- or well-child visit.
>
> Remember that every relationship has peaks and valleys. Your child's pediatrician is human, too, so give her a chance to make things better. Often differences of style or other difficulties can be worked out over time. On the other hand, if difficulties cannot be worked out and your child's needs are not being met, it may be reasonable to interview other pediatricians to find one who is a good fit for your family. After all, you'll be more likely to ask questions and share concerns if you feel comfortable with your pediatrician. If a doctor is not as approachable, you may be reluctant to discuss important issues that affect your child's care.

What's a Medical Home?

When we think of a home, we think of a building. But a medical home is not a physical structure. Instead, it's an approach to providing health care services that are accessible, family-centered, continuous, comprehensive, coordinated, compassionate, and culturally competent. The model was developed by the American Academy of Pediatrics and has since been adopted and promoted by other medical organizations. In this section, we'll look at what these terms mean and what you can do to help ensure that your child's medical team is living up to these standards. For more information, visit the National Center for Medical Home Implementation Web site at www.medicalhomeinfo.org/for_families.

Accessible

An *accessible* pediatric practice is one where the care you receive is provided right there in your community. The doctor and office staff should be available to you (at least by phone) after hours, on weekends, and during holidays, 24 hours a day, 365 days a year. At appointments, you and your child should be able to sit and talk with the pediatrician about any and all aspects of your child's care. The pediatrician and staff should be open and honest in their conversations with you while also listening to your concerns and questions. As a result of this relationship, you and your family should become well acquainted with the pediatrician and other members of the office staff such as nurses, nurse practitioners, and physician assistants, and you should feel comfortable asking them for information and resources for your child's needs. The office should help connect you to family support organizations in the community.

Being able to afford to care for a child with an ASD is also part of accessibility. In the event your pediatrician can no longer care for your child, the office should be able to accommodate you or refer you to another practice that provides the same kind of care.

Accessibility refers to physical access too. Being an accessible practice means that the facility is easy to enter and exit and meets the standards set by the federal Americans with Disabilities Act. If necessary and possible, the practice should be located near public transportation.

Family-Centered

In a *family-centered* medical home, the pediatrician is a familiar and trusted figure to the child and her family. But the family is regarded as the primary caregiver and source of support for the child. The relationship between the pediatrician and family is built on trust and mutual sharing of information. Both parties share in the decision-making process. The pediatrician should ask you about your concerns, what you've observed, and what might be the cause of these concerns. The information you provide should always be given careful consideration.

Meanwhile, your pediatrician should give you and your family all your treatment options in a clear, unbiased fashion. While sharing his expertise, the doctor should always respect you and your child as the experts in your child's care. If you pursue an option that is not in line with his recommendations, he should feel free to ask why and to share scientific evidence about the risks and benefits of that option. But he should also respect that decision, even if he doesn't agree with it.

Continuous and Comprehensive

When it comes to caring for a child with an ASD, consistency is important, especially for a child who does not like change. Ideally, the pediatric practice should have the same health care professionals taking care of your child from infancy to adolescence into young adulthood. And if your child sees a specialist, your pediatrician should review the report from that provider so that she can stay on top of all aspects of your child's care.

Although *continuous* care means your child should have access to a doctor 24-7, it does not necessarily mean that the doctor you talk to at midnight will be your primary care doctor. It's up to you to be familiar with the after-hours policies of your practice and to know who the other professionals are who may be involved in providing care.

When your child hits the teen years, continuous care may mean letting your child have a say in his own medical care. It can mean allowing him to take responsibility for his health care concerns, meet in private with his pediatrician, and take charge of his medications, appointments, and health records. (There is more about this in Chapter 11.)

Comprehensive care means the pediatrician is well-trained and able to manage all aspects of your child's care while also serving as an advocate for your child. Comprehensive care doesn't just mean handling illnesses. The doctor should also be involved in preventive medicine, which includes immunizations, growth and development, recommended screenings (such as hearing, vision, lead, cholesterol), and the proper supervision of care. The office staff and pediatrician should be open to advising parents on everything from health and safety, to parenting and psychosocial issues, to concerns about health insurance, Medicaid, and Title V state programs for children with special health care needs. If a family requires extra time to discuss these issues, the office should have a system in place to accommodate those needs.

Coordinated, Compassionate, and Culturally Competent

Pediatric care that is *coordinated* is central to the concept of a medical home. In a well-coordinated medical home, the pediatrician works closely with the family to develop an appropriate plan of care that meshes well with other health care practitioners, organizations, and agencies involved in your child's care. If others on your child's health care team make recommendations, the pediatrician should evaluate and interpret those recommendations for you.

A critical part of a coordinated care plan is the care notebook. The care notebook helps you keep track of all aspects of your child's care. Those same records should also be available in your doctor's office. We'll discuss more about the care notebook later in this chapter.

Compassion comes in the way the pediatrician and his staff treat you and your child. Concern can be verbal or nonverbal, but it should always be respectful and kind. Their concern should show up in the way they talk to you and listen to your concerns, and the amount of time and effort they put toward addressing your needs. The pediatrician should make an effort to really get to know your child and acknowledge the challenges that ASD imposes on your family.

Cultural competence refers to being sensitive to your values, beliefs, preferences, languages, and customs. The pediatrician and his staff should not judge you by your age, class, ethnicity, gender, race, sexual orientation, spiritual practice, or financial status. Of course it is up to you, the parent, to convey the values, customs, and preferences that are important to your family. For instance, if you are Jewish and eat a kosher diet, you cannot assume that your doctor knows this about you until you share this with him.

If English is not your primary language, your pediatric practice should seek out ways to communicate with you that are more effective, like enlisting a bilingual person to translate and provide written information in your primary language. Or you may want to hire a translator to join you on your doctor visits. Translators may be available through community or government agencies, colleges or universities, or local translation businesses. Make sure the translator understands the medical words and phrases that come up. A translator who has just learned to speak English may give incorrect information, which can be dangerous. It's

---

A PARENT'S STORY: JENNIFER

"As a single mom with 3 sons who have autism, I'm lucky to have a pediatrician who really listens. He is very patient and lets me carefully explain all of the minutiae of what is going on, no matter how insignificant the details may seem. Sometimes even the smallest details make sense to him and tip him off to something greater going on. He never makes me feel stupid for worrying or wondering or being tired or sad or confused. And he excuses me sometimes for the enormous burden that I face.

"I remember telling him one time just how hard homework was emotionally for my 7-year-old, who has an anxiety disorder. I told him I wished the school would just let him not do it because he was excelling academically. My pediatrician agreed with me but told me, 'I mostly agree that *you* don't need to do homework. Your days are hard enough, and your nights are hard enough.' So basically my pediatrician gave me a hall pass from homework and we were all happier at home. Everyone's anxiety went down after that.

"He makes my job easier because he trusts me. He knows that I have been working with all 3 of my sons so intensely, full-time, for 8 years now, and that I have been hands-on, 100% involved. So he trusts me to make the ultimate decision regarding their care and treatment.

"At the same time, we are truly a team. All of the decisions, from medication to changes in therapy, are made by both of us. I can decide to eliminate a speech therapy, for example, and explain to him why, and he trusts that I made the right call. He might give me reasons to reconsider, but he understands that my motivations are pure, that I am an educated mom, and that my desire to help my sons be successful comes from the same place of science and love that his decision to practice with this particular population did. We are both highly educated, empathetic, and practical people who want the best for my sons and are dedicated to doing whatever it takes to get them there. It feels like a blended personal *and* professional partnership. I trust him."

---

also best to hire translators who are at least 18 years old and who you trust. Telephone access to medical translators is available if none are readily accessible in person. To make sure information is accurately conveyed, you may ask the doctor to provide a written document of what you discussed. You'll be able to cross-check the accuracy of what the translator tells you.

Being a Good Parent Partner

Like any partnership, you need to devote time and energy toward the relationship you have with your child's pediatrician. After all, you are your child's primary caregiver, you know her better than anyone else, and the information you have about her is vital, whether it's pinpointing a diagnosis of autism or determining if a treatment is working. If you feel that you aren't being listened to, you may want to interview another physician who might be a better fit for your child and family.

To be a good parent partner, it's important to be an active player. If you choose, go to each doctor appointment armed with a list of questions and concerns. Be prepared to update your doctor about changes in your child's health and circumstances, such as changes in medications and treatments. Consider your pediatrician a key source of information, but always do your research and gather information from other sources too. Your pediatrician can also help you gain more knowledge by referring you to reputable Web sites, other parents, and books and articles (see Appendix A).

Don't be shy about telling your pediatrician of plans to ask other health care professionals for advice and second opinions. In fact, most pediatricians welcome a second opinion and may even give you a referral to another expert. And whenever possible, give your doctor feedback on how she is doing. Send a thank-you note for a suggestion she made that worked out well. Let her know when something doesn't go well too.

One of the most important things you can do is to keep good records of your child's medical and educational information. When several health care professionals are involved in a patient's care, it's easy for pieces of information to get overlooked or lost if a specialist doesn't send follow-up reports to your pediatrician. That's why your records are so important and warrant a discussion of their own.

Like any relationship, the way you conduct yourself can make a difference. If you want your doctor to listen to you, it's important that you listen to her. If you want to hear good news, make sure to share your good news too. Arrive on time so you help your doctor stay on schedule. Your child is but one patient in your pediatrician's busy day. If you need extra time for your visit, always let the scheduling staff know in advance.

Be clear with your pediatrician about how you want to work together and share in the decision-making process. Don't expect perfection from your pediatrician—doctors are human, too. If you're generally happy with your doctor and her practice, it may be worth enduring some difficult periods where you may not agree on treatment or philosophy.

Keeping Good Records: The Care Notebook

Tracking all your child's health and medical needs is a daunting task and can be especially overwhelming if you have a child with an ASD. Among all the therapies, health care specialists, and treatments, it can seem like a massive task just to stay on top of appointments, much less keep records of them. However, for the sake of your child's care, it's a task that should be done meticulously and regularly by you and your pediatrician.

That's where the care notebook comes in. A care notebook is an organizational tool that allows you to keep track of important information about your child's care. Having a comprehensive care notebook cements your role as the primary expert in your child's care. It is also a tool to help you communicate important information to your pediatrician. The care notebook should keep track of appointments and all aspects of your child's medical care as well as your child's special care needs, any community health services, records of his therapy, and issues at school, including the Individualized Education Program. More specifically, your care notebook should contain

- Routine doctor visits
- Immunization records
- Reports from specialists
- Medications, names, dosages, and frequency
- Laboratory tests and results
- Dietary changes
- Medical bills
- Insurance papers
- Types of activities of daily living that your child can do
- Notes about your child's social interactions, communication concerns, and ability to cope with stress

- Special transportation needs
- Early intervention services received
- Notes on conversations with school officials, including teachers
- Individualized Education Program/behavior intervention plan
- Transition plans
- Updated list of behavioral reinforcers or list of activities that can soothe or entertain your child

Bring your care notebook on all doctor visits, therapy sessions, and other appointments involving your child's care. You might also want to make a smaller version with the most vital health and medical information to take on vacation in the event of an unexpected illness.

Keeping the care notebook updated is an important task. Fill in details after each appointment and therapy session. Ask office staff for immunization records, doctor reports, laboratory test results, and any other information about your child that you require. For more information on how to build a care notebook, visit the National Center for Medical Home Implementation Web site at www.medicalhomeinfo.org/for_families.

The Doctor Visit

Going to a doctor, dentist, or any medical professional can be stressful for all children—adults too, for that matter—but for children with ASDs, these events can be downright distressing. The idea of someone touching your face or skin and even poking and prodding your body can cause enormous anxiety for a child who may already be extremely sensitive to stimuli.

For starters, a doctor's visit is a change in routine. It might mean pulling your child out of school early, interrupting a therapy session, or changing her meal schedule. The waiting room can be stressful too, especially if there are several other children and the wait is long.

The good news is, many practices are now becoming more sensitive to the needs of children with ASDs at appointments. So if you need to ask office staff for special accommodations, you should feel comfortable doing so. If your child needs time with the doctor to make her comfortable, ask if you can book a longer appointment. If sitting in the waiting room is too stressful, ask if you can wait in the car and be called on your cell phone when the doctor is ready. Many practices now are making these and other accommodations for families of children with special health care needs.

Of course, it's important that you relate your concerns to the doctor or dentist before you arrive at your visit. Tell office staff what bothers your child, but also share what comforts and interests him. This information can help staff make accommodations that will help you and your child have a better visit. Tell them about previous visits, what went well and what didn't.

It's also important to prepare your child for the visit. Talk to your child about what he can expect at a doctor or dentist visit. Look for books and videos that can show your child in a positive way what takes place. Try presenting appropriate behaviors in the form of a story (also known as social stories) with pictures about how to behave or react in a situation to teach your child. To make some of the procedures less frightening, practice some of them at home first. Take your child's temperature or blood pressure. Look inside his mouth with a tongue depressor. Peer inside his ears and nose. Listen to his heart with a stethoscope. Purchasing a toy doctor's kit beforehand can help him become familiar with the doctor's instruments. You might want to rehearse your visit in advance as well.

If your child has a hard time waiting, you might decide to book an appointment early in the day or immediately after lunch break, as these times tend to have shorter waits. You can also inform your pediatrician if you prefer to separate procedure visits from routine examinations. Some children with ASDs benefit from having a written schedule of procedures in the office on which items can be checked off as completed. This can be arranged with a nurse ahead of the visit and incorporated into a social story. If your child might need a vaccine or an uncomfortable procedure, talk to your pediatrician about how to best give that information to your child in a way that he can understand.

Sometimes, even with all your best efforts, a doctor's appointment can be challenging, especially if your child didn't get enough sleep the night before or if he is fearful about an impending immunization. In this case, you simply have to do the best you can to keep the appointment moving so you can reduce your child's time at the doctor's office. Enlist help from your spouse or a friend to accompany you. Come prepared with written questions.

A SUCCESSFUL VISIT: DR ROSENBLATT

"The good visit starts with an upbeat and welcoming staff who are sensitive to the child's special needs. This is followed by the doctor who takes time to bond with parent and child. The doctor should be flexible about the child's ability to handle the exam, which may take place on the parent's lap, the exam table, or standing up.

"The exam starts as simply as possible. I save what the child may perceive as the most frightening aspects of the exam until the end. I like to start by checking the hands and feet and then moving to the trunk and head. Whenever possible, I try to make a game out of the necessary parts of the exam. I allow the child to handle whatever instruments I use and practice the exam before it starts. Humor helps with some children but may irritate others.

"In certain circumstances no amount of charm or sensitivity will be able to calm a child's raging fear. In those situations I try to express my empathy and complete the exam as efficiently as possible.

"I try to make up for invading the child's personal space by declaring an end to the hard part of the visit and allow the child to be comforted by her parent. I will provide tissues to wipe away tears and drippy noses and may try helping the parent to console the child. Once the child is dressed and calmer, I may offer a special toy or activity for the child.

"After finishing my discussion with the parent, I check to see how the child says good-bye. From the children who respond to me, I will try to get a high five. If their response is forgiving, I will even try to get a hug. If they ignore or avoid my gesture, I will praise their bravery and say how proud I am of how they handled the exam. If the child is unable to understand what I am saying, I reassure the parent that we will try to minimize her child's discomfort in the future during necessary exams and procedures."

Bring a favorite toy or object that your child finds soothing. Do what you can to calm your child during the actual visit. You may choose to finish the appointment with a special reward, which will help your child associate doctor visits with something positive and enjoyable.

The Health Care Team

Because autism is a complex condition, it's possible that your child will have specialist doctors, in addition to your pediatrician, involved in his medical care. A great deal will depend on your child's particular health needs and concerns. Many of these doctors are pediatric specialists who work specifically with children in their areas of expertise. Here are some other types of health care professionals you may need.

- *Neurodevelopmental and developmental and behavioral pediatricians.* These specialists see children with developmental and behavioral concerns that may be signs of unusual brain function. Conditions commonly seen include ASDs as well as other disorders of development.
- *Neurologists.* Neurologists treat conditions affecting the nervous system, which includes the brain. Children who have seizures, headaches, and other symptoms related to the nervous system may be referred to neurologists for further testing.
- *Geneticists.* These physicians specialize in genetic disorders and conditions. They may ask questions about your medical history, take a family medical history, or perform a detailed physical examination. They may also order one or more tests to provide information or confirm a diagnosis. Geneticists might refer you to other specialists such as genetic counselors who provide information and support to patients and families affected by or at risk for genetic conditions.
- *Gastroenterologists.* These medical doctors treat health problems associated with digestion such as chronic or recurrent constipation and diarrhea, abnormal stool patterns, and abdominal pain.
- *Psychologists and psychiatrists.* These health care professionals work with patients to address challenging behaviors that result from mental health conditions such as anxiety, obsessive-compulsive disorder, and depression. While a psychologist has a graduate-level degree in psychology, a psychiatrist is trained in medical school. Psychiatrists focus more on medications, while psychologists generally are involved in specialized testing and behavioral therapies.
- *Registered dietitians or nutritionists.* Many children with ASDs are finicky eaters who may be at risk for nutritional deficiencies. A registered dietitian or nutritionist can help ensure your child gets the nutrients he needs.

When working with these other health care specialists, ask that any information about your child be sent to your pediatrician. Remember to ask them for their reports, and keep a detailed record of your visits. Be prepared to go to these appointments with all the information and questions you normally take to your pediatrician, such as names and dosages of drugs that your child takes.

Final Word

While you play the most critical role, your pediatrician is a key player in caring for your child. Together you should share one goal: to make sure your child receives the best medical care, therapies, and support available in your community. The key to meeting that goal is a solid relationship with your pediatrician, one that is built on mutual trust, respect, and understanding. In the next chapter, we'll go beyond your pediatrician and the rest of your medical team and take a look at the resources you may find in your community that will support you and your child.

CHAPTER 9

Services in Your Community

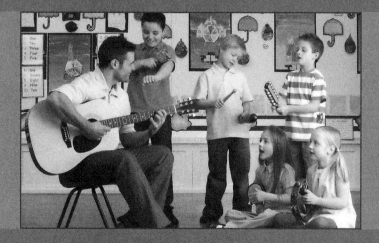

If you lived in Chicago and had a child with an autism spectrum disorder (ASD), you'd no doubt welcome a Web site like that offered by the city's premier parenting magazine, *Chicago Parent*. The site, www.chicagoparent.com, hosts a comprehensive list of services for children with ASDs, a list that includes everything from pediatric dental practices and therapy services, to parent support groups, to a Lego Club geared just for children with ASDs. The site is a wealth of information for parents looking for ways to support their children, learn about ASDs, and connect with other people, including other parents.

But not every city has a magazine like this, and not every magazine has such a detailed Web site. In fact, if you live in a rural community like Ellen does, you're not apt to find much. Ellen lives in a rural town in Utah, where there are few organizations dealing with issues surrounding autism. Fortunately, a local support group for parents of children with ASDs held a parents' night at her daughter's school, where she connected with the founder of the group. When that group was dissolved, she found a support group through a statewide organization that had local chapters. She also found resources through a program run by her state health department for children with special health care needs. It was simply a matter of looking, probing, and reaching out for Ellen to tap into the resources she needed to help her raise her son, who has autism.

Support for families with children who have ASDs comes in many forms. It may be educational, emotional, or financial. It may be practical or spiritual. In this chapter, we'll highlight the kinds of services a community might offer to children with ASDs and their parents and families. We'll also introduce you to some of the organizations involved in autism research and advocacy. Of course, it's impossible to cover every single type of service in every single community. But we hope this chapter will give you an idea of what's potentially available to you and ways for you to find these services. And if you're inspired, you may just want to launch something of your own to help other families in your own community.

Support Takes Many Forms

Whether you're looking to meet other parents who have a child with an ASD or you need information about the best therapies in your community, it helps to know about local organizations that assist children and families who are living with autism. The increase in the number of children with ASDs has given rise to a number of organizations as well as many state and local groups. For many people, these organizations become vital sources of information and support. Here are just a few.

Autism Science Foundation

The Autism Science Foundation (www.autismsciencefoundation.org) aims to support autism research by providing funding and other assistance to scientists and organizations conducting, facilitating, publicizing, and disseminating autism research. The foundation adheres to rigorous scientific standards and values because it believes that outstanding research is the greatest gift it can offer families.

The Autism Science Foundation also provides information about autism to the public and works to increase awareness of ASDs and the needs of individuals and families affected by ASDs. Through educational programs, the foundation also brings together parents and scientists. These opportunities help individuals with autism, their parents and siblings, and students and scientists to share their knowledge and expertise. Scientists benefit from hearing about the day-to-day experiences of families, and families hear directly about the latest in autism research.

Autism Society of America

The Autism Society of America (www.autism-society.org) is based in Bethesda, MD, and has chapters throughout the country. The group hosts a national conference, raises money for research, and strives to bring awareness to the issues surrounding autism. It also publishes a quarterly magazine and provides information about ongoing research.

Among its ventures is a partnership with AMC Theatres to provide sensory-friendly films every month for people with ASDs and other disabilities. During a sensory-friendly film, the movie auditoriums will be better lit and the sound will be turned down. Families will be allowed to bring their own gluten-free/casein-free snacks, and the presentation will have no previews or advertisements. Audience members will be free to get up and dance, walk, shout, or sing.

Autism Speaks

Autism Speaks (www.autismspeaks.org) raises money to fund research into the causes of, prevention of, and treatments for autism. The organization also strives to increase public awareness of autism and its effects on individuals, families, and society. Autism Speaks publishes documents and tool kits about various aspects of autism. It offers an online community where groups can chat about their concerns, ask questions, and share knowledge. An online resource library provides information about everything from safety products and assistive technology to books, magazines, and newsletters about autism.

Colleges and Universities

If you live in a town with colleges and universities that have robust education programs—especially those with a strong emphasis on special education—you may find support and programs on those campuses that benefit people with ASDs. Some colleges offer programs for children and families in the community as a way to teach students majoring in special education.

You can also find support and information through the Association of University Centers on Disabilities (AUCD). The AUCD is a membership organization that supports and promotes a national network of university-based interdisciplinary programs. Network members are made up of

- University Centers for Excellence in Developmental Disabilities (UCEDD), funded by the Administration on Developmental Disabilities, work with people who have disabilities, their families, state and local government agencies, and community providers on projects that provide training, technical assistance, service, research, and information sharing.
- Leadership Education in Neurodevelopmental and Related Disabilities (LEND) programs, funded by the Maternal and Child Health Bureau, are training programs usually found in a UCEDD that work with local university hospitals or graduate health care centers. Through LEND, children and their families can work with faculty and graduate students in their training to improve the health of children and adolescents with disabilities.

- Intellectual and Developmental Disabilities Research Centers, most of which are funded by the National Institute of Child Health and Human Development, strive to prevent and treat disabilities through biomedical and behavioral research. They also provide research training for scientists in different stages of their careers.

At least one of these programs exists in every state, and they are all part of universities or medical centers. They serve as a bridge between the university and community and bring together the resources of both. The UCEDD, for instance, have been involved in many issues important to families with children who have ASDs, such as early intervention (EI), health care, community-based services, education, and transition from school to work. The AUCD also has a Web site with a lot of information and news related to autism and other disabilities. You can find it at www.aucd.org.

National Dissemination Center for Children with Disabilities

Perhaps you're looking for information about EI services, or maybe you need resources to help your teenager transition into adulthood. The National Dissemination Center for Children with Disabilities (NICHCY) is a good place to start. The NICHCY offers information on disabilities and programs and services for infants, children, and youth with disabilities. It also has information on the Individuals with Disabilities Education Act and the No Child Left Behind Act that affect your child's education.

The NICHCY Web site, http://nichcy.org, can connect you to statewide organizations that can direct you to services in your community. The site also offers articles for parents on how to find services for your child, articles for teachers on how to discuss concerns about a child who may have a disability, and articles for employers on hiring people who have disabilities. You can find information about research and its importance in teaching children with disabilities.

The Power of Support Groups

Want to know the name of a good psychologist in your community? The most autism-friendly restaurant in your neighborhood? The best way to work with your school district? Talk to other parents. Most parents agree: one of the most helpful sources of information about ASDs—or any health condition for that matter—is other parents. You might meet these parents at school, at your doctor's office, or even out at a neighborhood playground. But one of the best places is in the context of a support group. A support group brings together people who are facing similar challenges, whether it's parenting a child who has an ASD, trying to lose weight, or overcoming an addiction.

A good support group is valuable on so many levels. For starters, it's a wealth of information. Here you'll meet other parents who have walked the same journey that you are now on. Like you, many have looked for medical experts to help their children, and many had the same questions that you do about therapies, medications, and schools. Tapping into a good support group is like finding a library filled with resources and information while also connecting with good friends.

Being surrounded by other people who are raising a child with an ASD helps you know what to expect while you move forward. It can be empowering and help you regain some sense of control over what may be a difficult situation.

But a support group does more than provide information. Run properly, it's also a tremendous source of emotional support. Learning that your child has an ASD can be tough, and you may experience a lot of challenging emotions as you go about the task of raising your child. Having a good support group gives you a place to unload those feelings of frustration, anger, and grief. It's also a great place to share your victories, happiness, and laughter with people who truly understand. In return, you will hear from other members who can offer you advice and share their own experiences. For many people, a support group can alleviate sadness and stress.

Of course, not all support groups are good ones. There may be some that are not aligned with your approach to your child's diagnosis and treatment. You also should be careful not to attend support groups in which you are not comfortable. Those that are dominated by talks of a cure or overrun by overly negative members may not be in your best interest. There are also groups that use high-pressure tactics to sell products or services or require high membership fees. And groups that prescribe medical advice or those that are judgmental may not be a good fit either.

If you want to join a support group, ask your pediatrician for names of local organizations. You can also talk with other health care professionals as well as friends, teachers, and therapists for ideas. (See also Appendix A.)

Online Support

In the age of the Internet, you can find almost anything on the Web, including support for families who have children with ASDs. Online support groups can be a great convenience if you don't have time to attend meetings or if you prefer the anonymity of the Internet. If you do choose to join an online group, know the terms of the Web site and how your personal information may be used. Steer clear of sites that aggressively market products or services. Be careful about giving out too much personal information, and understand that people may not be who they say they are. Here are a few you may want to check out.

Autism Support Network

According to its Web site, the Autism Support Network was founded with a simple mission: to connect, guide, and unite individuals and families faced with autism. In addition to a free online support community, the site provides a wealth of information about everything from diagnosis, therapies, and relationships to local resources in your state and community. It lists upcoming conferences, new research findings, and grant opportunities. The site also allows visitors to post questions to doctors. You can check out the network at www.autismsupportnetwork.com.

Autism Hangout

Autism Hangout is an online discussion forum that features news stories, blogs, videos, and information for parents of children with ASDs, as well as children and adults who have ASDs and other caregivers. Discussion forums cover everything from medications and therapies to stories about life with autism. The site also invites members to share information about products and services as well as reviews of books related to autism. Community members get to know and learn from one another. The Web site is www.autismhangout.com.

A DIFFERENT KIND OF SUPPORT: SERVICE DOGS

For children with autism spectrum disorders (ASDs) who are sensitive to sights and sounds around them, a service dog can be a soothing presence, a welcome companion and dependable guide. Well-trained dogs can even prevent a child from wandering or running away and help a child master social skills. There are many organizations that train these dogs to work specifically with children with ASDs, including Autism Service Dogs of America (http://autismservicedogsofamerica.com) and 4 Paws for Ability (www.4pawsforability.org).

Special Playdate

When your child has an ASD, giving her opportunities to learn social skills can be difficult. On Special Playdate, a free online service that links parents of children who have special needs, you can arrange playdates with other children who may have similar special needs. You can join the site and search for other parents by visiting www.specialplaydate.com.

Out 'n' About

Got a child who likes the water? If you live in Galveston, TX, you can enroll him in a sailing program called Heart of Sailing, designed just for people who have ASDs. Does your child love horses? In Elbert, CO, you can sign her up for therapeutic horseback riding at the Pikes Peak Therapeutic Riding Center. Got a young thespian in middle school? If you live in Plainview, NY, you can enroll him in Discover Theater.

The growing number of children with ASDs has spawned an industry of community services and businesses that cater exclusively to people with ASDs, which is good news for parents raising a child with autism. Whether it's art, Lego building, or martial arts, you can find organizations all over the country that will cater to your child's interests.

The surge in autism awareness has also inspired existing services to make special accommodations for children who have ASDs. Libraries, movie theaters, YMCAs, hotels, and theme parks are all offering special days or events for children with ASDs. At Walt Disney World, for instance, families whose children have disabilities such as ASDs can have special passes or wristbands that allow them to bypass the long lines that become so distressful for children with ASDs. Some restaurants now offer autism-friendly dining where employees are trained to be more patient and tolerant if children have challenging moments. At zoos that have become autism-friendly, you can find special maps and planning guides. Even hair salons are taking steps to make their services more accommodating to children with ASDs.

To assist with family travel, some hotel chains now have autism-friendly rooms with special door locks, shorter strings on the blinds, and a set of books in the room to create a homier feel. Corners of dressers and tables are covered to guard against unexpected falls, and doors may be equipped with alarms that warn you when someone tries to leave.

Churches and synagogues around the country are coming up with ways to cater to children with ASDs, too. Many of them have formed inclusion committees to discuss ways to incorporate the needs of people with ASDs into worship services. Some have created special services that are shorter in duration and allow children more freedom of movement and expression. Others have published religious books geared to children with ASDs.

A PARENT'S STORY: CARLY

"Our family is part of the Mormon faith. Our bishop is also the principal at the [school for children with special needs] my son Asher attends. Because he sees a lot of children who have autism, our bishop often has great ideas on how to make life better for these children.

"Recently, he ordered a swing for my son, which we attached to a basketball hoop in the gym at the church. He can swing on it to let out his stress and anxiety whenever he is overwhelmed during services. The bishop also asked 6 different people at church who are strong enough to handle my son to take turns supervising him every sixth Sunday. That way, none of them have him during church all the time. They take a turn every sixth week, and it gives my husband and me the opportunity to do the things at church that we need to do.

"It has been a fabulous program. The support, love, and service that people have given us in the church can never be fully repaid. It's a way to get lots of help without having to worry about the burden of finances. I'm very grateful for this program that my bishop came up [with] for us.

Getting the Services You Need

Obtaining these services has gotten easier over the years but may still require some phone calls and research. Here is how to access the most important ones your child will require.

Accessing Early Intervention

All states have an EI program for infants and toddlers with disabilities. The federally funded program was designed to help children younger than 3 years learn important developmental skills. The program also teaches families the skills they need to best work with their child. Exactly how the program is run varies from state to state.

Anyone can refer a child for EI services including the parent, the child's doctor, or a child care provider. Your child does not need a diagnosis to receive EI services. All you need for a referral is a concern that your child is experiencing a delay, though in some states, a diagnosis can provide your child with more specialized services.

Once your child is referred, a team of specialists will evaluate your child to determine if he qualifies. The team will write an Individualized Family Service Program (IFSP) that specifies the services your child needs. It also outlines goals, start and end dates of services, and steps to help your child and family transition to school services if your child still has developmental needs after he turns 3. A service coordinator will be assigned to your family to help coordinate services. Whenever possible, services will be administered in a place where your child is comfortable, such as his home or in child care.

Payment for EI services varies from state to state too. In some states, services are free of charge. In others, expenses are billed to the family's insurance plan. Some states charge according to the family's household income. Other states will provide services regardless of income. But all states must provide at least some services free of charge. These include screening for young children who have developmental or behavioral problems, testing to determine the types of services that are needed, coordination of services, and development, review, and evaluation of the IFSP.

You can get information about your state's EI program from your pediatrician, the state health department, or the local school district. You can also find information on the National Early Childhood Technical Assistance Center Web site at www.nectac.org.

Accessing School-Based Services

Once a child is 3 years old, she is able to receive services in the school with the help of the teaching staff. If a child has an ASD and it affects her performance in school, she is likely to qualify for school-based services. Gaining access to these services usually begins when a parent or member of the school's professional teaching staff refers a child for an evaluation to determine if there is a disability. Parental consent is needed before an evaluation can be done. If an evaluation reveals that the child has a disability, she may be eligible for special education services.

The degree of services, however, can vary widely. Some children have difficulties learning with regular curricula, even if they don't have a disability. For them, the first step may simply involve the classroom teacher informally trying different teaching approaches. The teacher may also do a response to intervention (RTI). An RTI involves consulting with other teachers, providing the child with more individual attention, or using other strategies to teach the child. All this can be done without additional testing of the child.

If a child needs more help than the classroom team can provide, a committee on special education may recommend using a Section 504 plan, which is named after the law that describes it. Section 504 guarantees that children with disabilities have equal access to an education, which means your child may receive accommodations and modifications that will support her ability to learn.

Some children, however, require an Individualized Education Program (IEP) tailored to their special needs. Individualized Education Programs are provided by the federal Individuals with Disabilities Education Act, which gives local schools funding for eligible students aged 3 to 21 years. An IEP outlines the educational program designed for your child and is written by the parents, the classroom teacher, a special education teacher, someone from the school system, and others. You can read more about IEPs in Chapter 5 or at www.wrightslaw.com.

A SPECIAL NOTE ON WANDERING

Wandering (also called elopement) is the tendency for a child to try to leave the safety of a responsible person's care or a safe area, which can result in potential harm or injury. Whether your child is at school, the local park, or even home, keep in mind that nearly half of all children with ASDs between the ages of 4 and 10 years will wander. In some cases, wandering continues well into a child's teen years. Children elope for a variety of reasons. They may want to escape a frustrating situation or sensory disturbances. Some wander off in pursuit of a special interest, such as trains, or to visit a place they enjoy, like the local park. Others elope for the simple pleasure of running or exploring.

Wandering is a serious safety concern for children with ASDs, who often lack the social and communication skills to return to safety. That's why parents and other caregivers must be made aware of the potential of wandering. If necessary, install security measures in your home such as dead bolts or alarm systems. If your child is wandering to get something or go somewhere, try to teach him other ways to obtain what he wants. Also, let your neighbors know that your child wanders. Vigilant neighbors can act as your eyes and ears and help reduce the risk of harm.

You can keep your child safe by having him wear a medical ID bracelet or tag that includes his name, telephone number, and any other important information. It's especially important to provide your child with some form of identification when you're on vacation, in case he wanders.

Of course, it's important to arm your child with basic safety skills. Teach your child to recite his name, address, and phone number. Get him in the habit of wearing his ID bracelet or tag whenever he goes out. Enroll him in swim lessons so he knows the basics of water safety. While you certainly want your child to explore and function in the world beyond his home, you also want him to be as safe as possible. For more information on wandering prevention and safety, visit the Autism Wandering Awareness Alerts Response and Education Collaboration at www.awaare.org.

All of these services are provided by your local school district at no additional cost. To find out more about school-based services, talk to your child's teacher or the special education staff at your child's school.

Finding Special Recreation Services

All children need physical activity to stay healthy, and children who have ASDs are no exception. Regular activity is important for teaching gross motor skills and exposing children to social opportunities. The key is finding the right programs for your child.

Often you can find these programs through your local parks and recreation department. Many communities now provide adaptive sports and recreation programs that are specifically designed for children with ASDs and other disabilities. These programs will take into account the unique ways your child learns and structure activities in ways that work best for your child. In fact, adaptive sports centers can be found around the country, offering everything from bowling and golf to skiing and outdoor adventure programs.

Some communities have specially designed parks and playgrounds for children with ASDs. If you're interested in finding parks designed specifically for children with ASDs, call your local parks and recreation department, the state parks department, or the US National Park Service. Although all children 16 years and younger are admitted to national parks for free, the US Geological Survey provides a free lifetime access pass for US citizens with a permanent disability that limits one or more major life activities. (Visit www.usgs.gov for more information.)

Even major theme parks now provide accommodations for children with ASDs and other special needs. Call in advance for information before you visit a park. The bottom line: children with ASDs are entitled to the same recreational activities that other children enjoy.

Final Word

These days, most communities offer a wealth of services for children with ASDs and their families. Seeking out these services can be richly rewarding for your child and for you and your family as well. Not only are the activities more accommodating to your child's special needs and more enjoyable for your child, but participating gives you the opportunity to meet other parents who are also raising a child with an ASD. We encourage you to look in your community for these kinds of services and to take advantage of the offerings.

Autism Champion: Denise D. Resnik

Denise D. Resnik suspected that something was wrong with her son Matthew. Soon after his first birthday he stopped speaking, started carrying around a plastic shovel, and no longer responded to his name. Tests showed his hearing was fine. "My mom gave me the book, *Let Me Hear Your Voice: A Family's Triumph Over Autism,* by Catherine Maurice, about a family's struggles and triumphs with autism," Denise recalls. "After the first few pages, I knew what we were dealing with."

Today, at 20 years of age, Matthew is a human GPS, a math whiz, and a young adult who eagerly helps out with chores like emptying the dishwasher, folding laundry, and taking out the trash. He also watches toddler movies to soothe himself, sneaks into his parents' bedroom several nights a week, and eats only a handful of different foods.

Like many other parents whose children have ASDs, Denise's life has been largely defined by her son's diagnosis. In 1997, she cofounded the Southwest Autism Research & Resource Center (SARRC) in Phoenix, AZ. What started as a mother's support group and coffee shop gathering has evolved into a nationally recognized nonprofit working with thousands of children, adults, and families affected by ASDs each year, along with physicians, educators, professionals, and paraprofessionals. With more than 85 employees, the organization provides lifetime support to individuals with ASDs and their families, and also advances research.

"Through the years, we've been growing up with our kids and doing our best to respond to the ever-increasing demand," says Denise, who owns a communications firm. "For us, it doesn't mean just directing individuals and families to SARRC for services, it's about being a catalyst and expanding support and options within the community through quality education, training, and evidence-based working models. It's also about advancing discoveries into the causes and most promising interventions."

But as Denise knows, autism doesn't end in childhood, and the needs of adults are on the rise. SARRC is a driving force behind Advancing Futures for Adults with Autism, a consortium of more than a dozen regional and national organizations working to "create meaningful futures for adults with autism that include homes, jobs, recreation, friends and supportive communities."

Denise is convinced that with the proper support, adults with ASDs are capable of becoming engaged citizens. "Like most parents, my husband and I continue to wrestle with pressing concerns like where Matt lives as an adult," she says. "How will he continue to progress and become a productive, contributing member of our community? How can we be assured he'll be safe, secure, and accepted when we're no longer here to watch over him?"

Denise envisions Matthew living in a home with friends, pursuing his education and skill development, working someplace where he is valued, and continuing his volunteer work.

"Matt is one of the hardest working young adults I know," says Denise. "With his work ethic, results-driven focus, and kindness, he'll be an excellent employee and a very good neighbor."

CHAPTER 10

Accessing Care

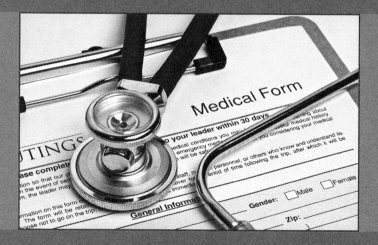

Annabelle lives in Wisconsin where her son with autism has received financial assistance for therapy sessions. Because of his disability, her son qualified for waivers that helped pay for camps, social skills training, and in-home therapy. Household income wasn't a factor. All it took was some perseverance and research for Annabelle to secure the money.

Let's face it: raising a child with an autism spectrum disorder (ASD) is expensive. Research published in 2006 by Michael Ganz at the Harvard School of Public Health has shown that the cost of caring for someone with autism is $3.2 million over a lifetime. Children who have ASDs typically require more visits to the doctor's office, an array of therapy services, and multiple medical treatments. Between the ages of 3 and 7 years, behavioral therapies alone can rack up $32,000 or more in costs. Indirect costs include all the lost time and wages by parents who must take time off from work to care for their child.

For some people, affording the care can be a major struggle and even a hurdle to securing the help their child needs. In this chapter, we will take a look at the various sources of financial assistance available to you, be it government programs, grants from private organizations, or insurance coverage for ASD services. We'll also take a look at the laws that govern your access to these services so you know what you are entitled to receive. With a little initiative and persistence you may be able to access the kind of resources that Annabelle was able to obtain for her son.

Government Programs

Financial assistance is available from federal and state government programs, but each has its own set of rules, regulations, and procedures.

Supplemental Security Income

Supplemental Security Income (SSI) is an important source of financial support for low-income families who have children with special health care needs and disabilities. According to the US Social Security Administration (SSA), there were 1.2 million children younger than 18 years who were receiving SSI in 2009. In the majority of states, being eligible for SSI qualifies your child for the state Medicaid program, which provides access to health care.

Supplemental Security Income is administered by the SSA, funded by the federal government, and in some places also receives state support.

To qualify, a child must have a medically determined physical or mental impairment or a combination of impairments that result in marked and severe functional limitations. The disability has to have lasted or be expected to last at least 1 year.

To determine if your child's disability makes her eligible for SSI, your child will need to be evaluated. This process is handled by Disability Determination Services (DDS). Every state has its own name for the agency that handles the DDS, but they are all overseen by the SSA. To make a decision, a disability examiner and medical or psychological professional will gather information from parents, physicians, hospitals, psychologists, teachers, schools, social workers, friends, relatives, and anyone else acquainted with the child who may provide information about her impairments and functioning. Medical records from your child's pediatrician are especially important for reaching a decision. The disability examiner and medical or psychological professional must then determine if the disability is in fact "severe" enough to qualify for SSI services.

Eligibility and the actual amount of financial support you receive depend on family income, whether it's a 1- or 2-parent household, how many siblings there are, and financial assets. A child may be denied SSI if the child herself is engaged in "substantial gainful activity," meaning she's working and earning more than a certain amount of money. The total figure that is allowed is determined annually. Supplemental Security Income can be an important source of support and health benefits for young adults in transition. For more information about SSI, contact the SSA at 800/772-1213 or check out its Web site at www.ssa.gov.

Social Security Disability Insurance

Supplemental Security Income is not to be confused with Social Security Disability Insurance (SSDI), which is given to any unmarried child younger than 18 years (or between 18 and 19 years of age and still in high school) whose parents are disabled or retired and receiving Social Security retirement or disability benefits. Unlike SSI, the SSDI program is funded through Social Security, using monies collected through the Federal Insurance Contributions

---

FAST FACT

Title V of the Social Security Act created maternal and child health programs throughout the United States. Children who qualify are eligible for health care services as part of the provision for children with special health care needs. These programs are usually managed by state health agencies and come by many names, including Children's Special Health Services and Children's Medical Services. Most of these programs are offered through clinics, private offices, hospital outpatient and inpatient treatment centers, or community agencies.

If your child does not get SSI, you may still be able to get help from one of these programs. Contact your state or local health department, social services office, or a local hospital and find out how you can contact your local program for children with special health care needs.

Act. There are no income and asset limits to receive SSDI, but payments are based on the parents' employment history and amount they have paid into Social Security.

An adult disabled before age 22 may be eligible for a child's benefits if a parent is deceased but worked long enough under Social Security, or is currently receiving retirement or disability benefits. An adult child can also receive SSDI benefits if the child received dependent benefits on the parents' Social Security earnings before the child was 18. An adult receiving SSDI benefits becomes eligible for Medicare after a 2-year waiting period. To qualify, an adult must have an appropriate medical diagnosis and be able to demonstrate that his disability interferes with his ability to secure gainful employment.

If your child is 18 years or older, his disability will be evaluated in the same way it would be for any adult. The decision is made by your state's DDS.

Applying for Supplemental Security Income or Social Security Disability Insurance

To apply for these programs, you need to visit your local Social Security office or call the toll-free number 800/772-1213. If you are applying for SSI payments for your child, you should bring her Social Security number and birth certificate with you. If you are applying for SSDI benefits for your child, bring along your own Social Security number as well as your child's Social Security number and birth certificate.

The SSA will contact your doctors to obtain your child's medical records, but you can help by providing as much information as possible about your child's medical condition. It's not necessary for you to request information from your child's pediatrician and other doctors, but it does help if you can provide as much information as possible about your child's medical condition, records of her doctor and hospital visits, and patient account numbers that will help the SSA obtain her medical records. If you do have copies of any medical reports or information, you can also present those to the SSA.

You may be requested to bring other documents and information too. For instance, if you're applying for SSI for a child younger than 18, you will need tax records and employment papers to show your income and assets as well as those of your child. The SSA may also ask you to describe how your child's ASD affects her ability to function on a daily basis, and ask you for the names of teachers, family members, and child care providers. You may want to bring along any school records to your interview with the SSA.

Many communities now have special arrangements with medical providers, social service agencies, and schools to help the SSA obtain the evidence it needs to process your claim. But anything you do that helps the SSA get the records it needs will help it process your application more quickly.

Home and Community-Based Service Waivers

Some individuals may qualify for services and supports through the Home and Community-Based Services (HCBS) Waiver program, also known as section 1915(c) of the Social Security Act, which was signed into law in 1981. Home and community-based services are provided by state Medicaid programs and funded through a combination of federal and state funding. The waivers allow states to waive certain Medicaid restrictions, such as income, so individuals can obtain medically necessary services in their home and community that might otherwise be provided in an institution, as the section 1915(c) program requires an individual to meet institutional level-of-care requirements. Services that are covered help support people with disabilities, including ASDs, and are designed to help them live more independent lives. The waivers allow states to cover an array of home and community-based services, such

SPECIAL NEEDS TRUST

If your child receives a substantial amount of money as a gift or through another person's will, you may wish to create a document called a special needs trust (SNT) (also called a supplemental care trust). It is a legal tool that ensures that inheritance money is available to your child when he needs it. The SNT provides for the needs of your child without disqualifying him from benefits received from government programs like Supplemental Security Income (SSI) and Medicaid. If the money is left in a traditional will, the person must use that money first for living expenses and health care until the money is depleted. To be sure that needed government assistance continues, assets must be placed in the trust and set up correctly.

Money placed in the SNT can only be used for items and services not covered by Medicaid, SSI, or other state or federal funds, but funds cannot be given directly to the person with a disability. Instead, it must be given directly to a third party to pay for goods and services to be used by the person with a disability. The trust may be used for expenses such as transportation, materials for a hobby or recreational activities, computers, and vacations. The funds cannot be used for food, shelter, or clothing.

The money in the trust can be invested and earn unlimited money. Assets and earnings belong to the trust, not the child. Parents can establish and fund the trust and act as trustees while they are alive, or the trust can be written so that is established by the parents' will and starts to function after the parents' death. There are numerous advantages to establishing a trust early, even before your child turns 18.

If you wish to create an SNT, make sure to contact an experienced lawyer. Ask your pediatrician for a referral or contact your local bar association. You may also find help from related nonprofit organizations.

as respite care, modifications to the home environment, and family training, that may not otherwise be covered under a state's Medicaid plan.

A small number of states even offer autism-specific 1915(c) waivers. The ages of the children who can receive waivers vary by state, as do the types of services that are covered. In Maryland, for instance, the Medicaid waiver provides intensive individual support services, respite care, and other services. But the program, as in most HCBS waivers, is only available to a fixed number of individuals. In states without an autism waiver, individuals may be able to qualify for services under another program. In some instances HCBS has created access to highly specialized services for children and adults with ASDs.

In general, HCBS waivers fund specific programs and services and do not directly give funding to individuals. But some states have established self-directed programs that allow individuals to use the funds to purchase the services they need themselves and hire and fire the staff they want. Generally, the waiting period for services can be long, sometimes taking several years.

The best thing you can do is to call your local or state Medicaid office as soon as your child is diagnosed with an ASD to begin the process. You should ask your pediatrician for the name of the agency that handles HCBS. Once your child is approved for funding, you will work with a case manager to create an annual service plan that pinpoints the exact supports you require. Depending on your state, the waiver may apply to medical equipment, home remodeling for safety concerns, and therapy services. The case manager oversees your plan and makes sure that you are receiving quality services, while ensuring that you are comply-ing with the rules as well. From time to time, your case manager may call you and make sure your needs are being met.

The process for submitting a waiver application is different in each state just as the types of services available to you will vary depending on where you live. For more information, con-tact your state or county offices of the departments of Health and Human Services, Mental Health, and Intellectual Disability, or the state developmental disabilities organization.

Tax Equity and Financial Responsibility Act of 1982

Some states offer Medicaid coverage to certain disabled children through a program called the Tax Equity and Financial Responsibility Act of 1982, also known as TEFRA. This might also be referred to as a Katie Beckett waiver in your state, named for a girl whose mother helped spearhead passage of TEFRA. The Tax Equity and Financial Responsibility Act pro-vides Medicaid coverage to children who are severely disabled but whose parental income would otherwise disqualify them. Funding is intended to benefit children whose disabilities may require care in an institution but whose family has chosen to care for them at home. Some states such as Pennsylvania and New Hampshire offer programs similar to TEFRA. Again, you should contact your state Medicaid agency to determine if TEFRA is offered.

Government Health Insurance

Most people who have full-time jobs have health insurance. Perhaps your insurance covers your child's many needs for his ASD. But if you don't have private health insurance, you may be able to get help from state and federal government programs. Here are a few programs to look into.

Medicaid

Medicaid is a joint program of the federal and state governments that provides medically necessary services to low-income families and children who meet specific eligibility requirements. The numbers of children who have special needs and receive Medicaid has risen significantly in recent years. For many eligible children, Medicaid is often their sole source of health insurance. In some cases, individual participants may be asked to share in the cost for certain services.

Unlike Medicaid HCBS waiver services, Medicaid state plan services are typically restricted to covered services, and for children include services covered under the federal Early Periodic Screening, Diagnosis and Treatment (EPSDT) program, which mandates basic preventive and therapeutic health services that are deemed appropriate and necessary for children. Some states may elect to qualify school-based personnel as service providers. Each state sets its own guidelines and determines who is eligible and which optional services are covered.

To understand what your state offers, visit your state's Medicaid Web site, the Centers for Medicare & Medicaid Services (CMS) Web site at www.cms.gov, or the CMS Medicaid-specific Web site at www.medicaid.gov. You can also get information from other parents and disability organizations; see Appendix A for suggestions.

Children's Health Insurance Program

The Children's Health Insurance Program, also known as CHIP, provides free or low-cost health insurance to children from working families with incomes that are too high to qualify them for Medicaid but too low for them to afford private health insurance. The program covers prescription drugs, vision care, hearing assistance, and mental health services and is available in all 50 states and the District of Columbia. It also covers routine checkups, immunizations, hospital care, dental care, and laboratory and x-ray services. Children get free preventive care, but low premiums and other services may require you to pick up some of the costs.

Each state creates its own CHIP and determines eligibility, benefits, premiums, and application and renewal procedures. In general, in 2011, a family of 4 with an annual household income of up to $44,100 a year was eligible for coverage.

To find out more about CHIP in your state, contact your state Medicaid agency. You can also get information on the Internet at www.insurekidsnow.gov or by calling 877/KIDS NOW (543-7669).

Private Health Insurance

Most private insurance companies do not cover therapies for autism. Sadly, some private insurance policies even contain outright bans on autism treatments. Some policies cover some aspects of care but almost always refuse to pay for the behavioral and developmental treatments that are the cornerstones of effective autism therapy.

However, some states do have insurance laws that require private health insurance companies to cover autism treatments such as applied behavior therapy, occupational therapy, and speech-language therapy. As of early 2012, autism coverage by private insurance plans was mandated in more than half of the states. In addition, state laws that require insurance coverage of services for children in need of habilitative care (including treatment for autism) existed in just 2 states—Illinois and Maryland.

If you don't live in one of these states, don't automatically assume that your child's services and therapies are not covered. You may be able to obtain coverage if your insurance company

---

PRIVATE INSURANCE UPDATE

The recently enacted Patient Protection and Affordable Care Act contains several provisions within private insurance reform that benefit families of children with disabilities. These include

- Eliminating lifetime and annual caps on benefits

- Guaranteeing coverage through elimination of preexisting condition denials

- Expanding dependent coverage up to age 26

Once exchanges are established by 2014, benefits for health plans must include chronic disease management, behavioral health treatment, habilitation and rehabilitation services and devices, and oral and vision care. The scope of each of these benefits, though, is yet to be defined.

A PARENT'S STORY: NORA

"Last summer, my daughter Rory received $1,500 from the Jewish Social Services Agency to pay for weekly horseback riding lessons. Now I'm waiting to hear about my application to receive money from the Low Intensity Support Services [LISS] program through The Arc, which serves people with developmental disabilities in Maryland. The LISS money would help us pay for a day camp this summer and would amount to $595 for 2 weeks. I had to fill out applications for both grants, but the effort was well worth it.

"I learned about these funding sources from the parents in Rory's class. They've also helped me find sensory-friendly movie theaters, good places for haircuts, and support groups. The best sources of autism information of any kind, I've found, are other parents."

---

is based in one of the states that has an autism insurance mandate or by showing that the treatments are medically necessary. And if you are receiving services for another condition besides autism, you may be able to secure coverage by stating that problem as the reason for the services.

Assistance From Private Organizations

Numerous organizations around the country offer scholarships, family grants, and other types of funding for people with ASDs to help pay for expenses related to autism. Finding these organizations takes some digging, but if you don't mind doing the work, you may be able to find funding. The Autism Relief Foundation, for instance, offers grants of $300 to $1,800 for medical services, autism therapies, and summer camps. The United Healthcare Children's Foundation provides financial assistance to children who have private health insurance but whose plans don't cover all their needs.

When you apply for a scholarship or grant, read everything carefully. Make sure you satisfy all the requirements and send in the information it needs. Check to be sure that you fit the criteria before you even put pen to paper. Pay close attention to deadlines. Keep a copy of whatever you send in. If you don't get funding the first time, you can use that information to apply again in the next cycle.

MONEY MATTERS

We'd love to send our daughter to a summer camp for children who have autism, but the camp is expensive. Where can we get help?

Autism Speaks offers scholarship funds through the Baker Summer Camp Program. The program offers up to $3,000 in scholarships to eligible campers at selected camps. All camps in the United States that provide a summer program to financially disadvantaged individuals with autism were eligible to apply. In 2010, 280 camps submitted scholarship grant applications. Money was then distributed to more than 330 campers at 51 camps across the country.

My sister's family was just in a hurricane, and they are having a hard time affording their son's autism services. Can they get any help?

Financing treatments and therapies for ASDs is already expensive, and paying for them in the face of a natural disaster can break the bank. Your sister may qualify for help from Autism Cares, a consortium of major autism organizations that have come together to support individuals with ASDs and their families during natural disasters and other catastrophic life events. The organization helps cover the costs of living expenses such as housing, utilities, car repair, child care, funeral expenses, and other essential items. For more information, check out the Autism Cares Web site at www.autismcares.org.

Autism Champion: Lorri Unumb, JD

When Lorri Unumb's son Ryan was diagnosed with an ASD, his therapies added up to $75,000 a year out of pocket. But Lorri knew she had no choice. "My husband and I are both lawyers and, compared to most lawyers, we don't make a lot of money, but we made enough to sacrifice one salary to get therapies for Ryan," she recalls. They also moved to a less expensive house and began cutting costs.

Lorri, who also has 2 typically developing sons, was acutely aware that other families weren't so lucky. "I'd go to these support groups with other moms, and they didn't have an extra salary to sacrifice," she says. "It drove a stake through my heart thinking how difficult it must be. It just wasn't fair. They couldn't afford therapy for their child, but they were still paying insurance premiums every month."

The injustice inspired her to pursue changes in insurance coverage for ASD services in South Carolina where she lives. Lorri recruited other parents, began visiting legislators, and wrote a bill in 2005.

The battle wasn't easy. "When you're an autism parent, many days, it's all you can do to get through bath time and bedtime before you collapse," she says. "The last thing you have energy for is to battle insurance companies."

In 2007, the law was passed. Ryan's Law—named for her son and in memory of her father, Ryan Shealy, a former state legislator—requires insurance coverage for ASD services and served as a catalyst for nationwide ASD insurance reform.

"In many ways autism has been a blessing in my life," Lorri says. "I can't say I'm glad my child has autism. At the outset all I wanted to do was figure this out and grieve. Now I have a different perspective. I can appreciate the way autism has changed my life and given my life meaning. I'm almost 43, and I see people around my age struggling to find meaning and purpose in this life. That's something I don't have to struggle with. It brings a certain fulfillment, and for that, I'm grateful."

CHAPTER 11

Adolescence and Beyond

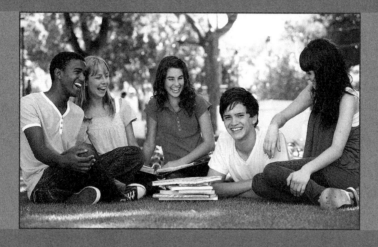

When her son Paul was first diagnosed with autism in 1994, Charlotte didn't know if Paul would ever ride a bike or talk on the phone. As for herself, she decided to put her journalism career on hold to care for her son and spent hours driving him to various forms of therapy. During his early teens, she homeschooled him for 2 years.

Growing up was scary for Paul, now 20. Unlike most teenagers, Paul didn't want a cell phone. He didn't want to carry a wallet, and he didn't want a job. Girls? They terrified him.

In his late teens, all that began to change. He had his first girlfriend, landed a job bagging groceries at the local supermarket, and graduated from high school. But his parents were still uncomfortable with the idea of Paul moving into a precollege independent living situation. "We feared he'd spend too much time alone," Charlotte said. "We weren't sure he'd advocate for himself."

Charlotte and several other parents banded together and began discussing all the challenges that confront children with autism once they turn 18 and become adults. They decided to do research into their options and to share the information. Together, 3 of the families decided to create a transition program. They rented a house, hired a director, and assigned each boy to a bedroom. The goal of the program is to train the boys to live independently and to master skills like banking, cooking, cleaning, shopping, and navigating public transportation. They also do social skills training, visit a gym twice a week, and do yoga 5 days a week. Recently, Paul and one of his housemates began taking driver's education in the hopes of getting their driver's permits.

Charlotte has since decided to formalize the program for other young adults with autism. And Paul is making plans to attend a boarding school for young adults with disabilities and take classes. He hopes to become an artist someday. "It blows my mind to see the distance he has travelled," Charlotte says of her son. "It literally inspires me every day."

Moving from childhood into adolescence is a major step in any child's life. These are the years when your child starts thinking about his future, what he'll do for a job, where he'll live, and how he'll live as an adult. These are also the years of significant physical changes, as hormones shift and your child slowly evolves into an adult. And then there are the changes in social expectations as friendships become more central and the possibility of dating looms.

As any parent of a teenager will tell you, adolescence is a critical turning point. Your child is approaching young adulthood, and along with it comes a host of physical, mental, and emotional changes. The child who has an autism spectrum disorder (ASD) will experience changes as well, with some, like Paul, making great strides in their social skills and experiencing a lessening of their symptoms.

In this chapter, we'll give you an idea of what many adolescents with ASDs may experience during these years and what you can do to help promote a smooth transition from adolescence through the teen years and into adulthood. We'll take a look at the all-important transition plan as your child begins to look forward to his adult life in the community. We'll also discuss some of the practical steps you can take to help your child live more independently. In addition, we'll explore some of the physical, emotional, and social changes that are occurring that may affect your child's well-being.

As we address these issues, keep in mind that transition from childhood to adulthood will be unique for each child. For example, children with ASDs and intellectual disability may have different goals and expectations than those without intellectual disability. This is all the more reason to work in partnership with your pediatrician to make sure these changes are thoughtful and respectful of each child's level of development.

The Transition Plan

Remember the Individualized Education Program (IEP) that laid out all the details of your child's education while he was in elementary school? As you may recall, the IEP was created as part of the Individuals with Disabilities Education Act (IDEA), which gives your child access to special education services. One of the basic goals of IDEA is to prepare students for employment and independent living. To that end, the law requires that all children who receive special education services have a transition plan in place by the time they turn 16 years old. Ideally, the process should begin at age 14. Once your child turns 21, he is no longer eligible for special education services offered under IDEA, but he may be eligible to receive services until that time.

In short, the transition plan is the road map that could help prepare your child to participate as much as possible in community life once school is completed. And those individuals with ASDs have a range of options once their education is completed. Some may benefit from a highly structured vocational or day program, while others may pursue employment in a sheltered, supported, or competitive setting. Still others may wish to pursue some form of higher education or trade school before joining the workforce. The most important thing is that for many people, adults with ASDs included, having a job helps define and give meaning to their lives. The transition plan outlines your child's specific goals as he prepares for adulthood. It should also address his health care needs, job and career options, community participation interests, and plans for continuing education.

The thought of your adolescent getting a job might seem too far in the future for you to contemplate right now. It might also be difficult to imagine your child holding down a job. But in reality, adolescence is a good time to start talking to your child about what he wants to do in the future. You might want to start by discussing different jobs and skills that are of interest to him. You may want to talk about people he knows who are going to college, getting a job, or living on their own. Some adolescents may find the prospect of striking out on their own rather frightening. To make the discussions less anxiety-ridden, you may want to set aside a time and day every week to discuss your child's future. Knowing that it's on his schedule will help him plan what he wants to discuss and ease his anxieties about the discussion.

In drafting the transition plan, you need to take into account your child's learning capacity and then consider several questions, such as

- What does your child like to do?
- What are your child's dreams and goals in life?
- What is your child able to do? What are his strengths?
- What does your child need to explore?
- What does your child need to learn to reach his goals?
- Does your child have future education goals?
- How do you and your child feel about him getting a job?
- What are some possible job options for your child?
- What are the skills and supports needed for a job?

- What kinds of transportation does your child have available to him?
- Where will your child live?
- How will your child get health insurance?
- Are supports necessary to encourage friendships?
- Do people in the community know your child?
- Does your child need supports to structure time for recreation?
- Does your child have a system for communicating that is effective?
- Does your child require additional strategies to improve his communication?
- What other supports might your child need?

When creating the transition plan, it's important to consider your child's existing support systems, financial planning needs, long-term care needs, and access to community, state, and federal resources. You should also take into account the kind of support he has from family members, including siblings. The plan you ultimately create should be outcome-oriented and based on your child's strengths and areas of need. It should set realistic goals and specific strategies for meeting those goals, especially if your child has challenges that need to be addressed. It should also be laid out on a timeline so the plan has details about when important events are coming and which resources are needed to address goals.

Keep in mind that the transition plan is a work in progress, one that should be revisited several times a year. Over time, your child will continue to grow and learn, and the transition plan should be adjusted accordingly. But start the process early so you can tap into the educational resources available to you. And make sure to include others, such as your child's educators and therapists, in the process.

Whatever you do, make sure your child is involved in the process of creating the transition plan as much as possible. The process can be a way to develop your child's self-advocacy skills, which will become increasingly important as he ages. Of course, different children will be able to participate at different levels. Some, because of challenges with cognitive skills and communication, may need more assistance than others. The important thing is that your child should be encouraged to participate in planning about the future to the fullest extent possible. Ideally, your child should know about his disability and be able to discuss it with others. (See "Discussing an Autism Spectrum Disorder Diagnosis With Your Child" on pages

---

FAST FACT: WHO ELSE IS INVOLVED?

Many people may be involved in your child's transition planning, including

- Your child

- You and other caregivers

- Special education teachers

- Other teachers

- School administrators

- Therapists and other service providers

- Representatives of outside agencies that may support your child after the transition

- Other individuals who can support your child

---

106 and 107 in Chapter 5.) He should be able to tell others about any special accommodations he needs.

Boosting Your Child's Self-Advocacy

Every parent wants her child to be able to speak up on her own behalf, whether it's ordering a meal in a restaurant or standing up for herself when she thinks she's been treated unfairly. Self-advocacy is the ability to take responsibility for your choices and decisions and to express your needs and ask for help. These are all vital skills that a child acquires gradually over time. The ability to advocate for yourself is essential to any child's growth and development.

For most of your child's life, you may have been her primary advocate, which means you've made many decisions for her. You chose the therapies she required, told her when to get out of bed, and sent her to activities that you thought suited her personality and interests. But as your child gets older, the goal is to have her learn to advocate for herself to the extent that she can, which means assessing a situation, realizing that something requires action, and speaking up about what she needs or wants. It means knowing her rights and responsibilities and using the proper resources to reach a decision. For children who have ASDs, self-advocacy also means being aware of their disability and being able to communicate it to others verbally or through the use of pictures, written words, or gestures. Although all children with ASDs may not be able to fully advocate for themselves, the goal should be to work to achieve the highest level possible.

Like everything else you have taught your child, teaching her about self-advocacy will require patience, time, and the understanding that it's a process, not a quick lesson. Encouraging self-advocacy starts with giving your child choices in life, from the cereal she eats for breakfast to what shirt to wear. As she gets older, you will be able to give her even more choices. When should she clean her room? What time should she go to bed on a Friday night? What activities should she participate in?

Breaking down the process of decision-making into simpler steps can help too. According to the Wisconsin Department of Public Instruction handbook, *Opening Doors to Self-Determination Skills: Planning for Life After High School*, these steps are

1. What is the decision you need to make?

2. What decisions could I make? (In other words, what are the possibilities from which to choose?)

3. Evaluate each choice. What are plusses and minuses of each choice?

4. Pick the best choice. Describe which choice you think is best for you.

5. Evaluate. Did you make the best choice for you?

Carefully considering decisions in a step-by-step fashion will help your child become more aware of the many choices she faces and better understand her options. Eventually, making decisions will come more easily and be less of a regimented process.

When and how do I tell my child he has an autism spectrum disorder?
Talking with your child about his diagnosis is a process, not a one-time conversation. The whole concept of "having an autism spectrum disorder" is a lot to take in. It's going to take some time, with new questions asked and deeper understanding gained as your child matures. There is no exact age or time that is correct to tell a child. Your child's personality, abilities, and social awareness are all factors to consider in determining when he is ready for information about his diagnosis. For example, a parent may decide to talk about autism spectrum disorders when the child begins asking questions such as, "Why am I different?"   (For more information, see "Discussing an Autism Spectrum Disorder Diagnosis With Your Child" on pages 106 and 107 in Chapter 5.)

Encouraging Daily Living Skills

All your child's life, you've been gently nudging him toward greater independence to the best of his ability. And hopefully you've been doing that with an eye toward his future and the knowledge and abilities he will need to navigate his way through the world. If you haven't done that, now is the time to really build these skills. As your child reaches adolescence, it becomes more important to think about the skills he'll need to live and work independently, now and in the future. For instance, it may be important to teach him how to ride public transportation and to show him how to use money for purchases.

To encourage your child to absorb these skills for daily living, keep in mind that people learn best when skills are taught in the setting where they are used. It's best to apply these lessons using actual objects and to do it at the time these tasks are most often performed. For instance, if you want to teach your child how to use money, take him to a store and teach him how to pay for something. Don't only use play money at home. If you want to teach your child to wash his face before bed, give that lesson at bedtime, not in the middle of the day. It's also important to know that children with ASDs learn best when they are motivated to obtain something or gain access to an activity that they highly desire.

Medical Concerns During Adolescence

For the most part, the medical issues of childhood improve during the teenage years, but there can be some new challenges. Puberty is tough, even among children with typical development. In children with ASDs, the body changes that occur with puberty can create new challenges. Adolescence is a peak time for children with ASDs to develop seizures, the other time being the preschool years. (For more information on medical issues in a child with an ASD, such as sleep difficulties and gastrointestinal problems, see Chapter 3.)

Likewise, a child with an ASD who has tics may find his tics worsening on entering adolescence. If your child has been an extremely finicky eater, he may experience difficulty keeping up with the growth demands of adolescence. It is important to continue to work with your pediatrician on these and other medical conditions because treating them will help your child prepare to meet the challenges of adolescence.

Adolescence also is the time to start preparing for the transition of your child's medical care to an adult health care professional. National professional organizations, including the American Academy of Pediatrics (AAP), recommend that families of children with disabilities begin planning and setting long-term goals for the future health care needs of their children at age 12 years. (See Chapter 10, page 205, for information on the Patient Protection and Affordable Care Act that addresses health care needs of individuals with disabilities.) A health care transition plan should be developed with health care professionals by the time a child is 14 years old. Starting early allows for time to teach self-management skills and prepare children and families for the choices they will need to make.

It is important to plan this transition with your child's pediatrician well in advance to avoid lapses in meeting your child's health care needs. Many families have found it difficult to find adult providers with experience in treating adults with ASDs. Your pediatrician can help you in the process of identifying adult primary care practitioners and specialists who will be part of the adult medical team. Once that happens, a plan can be made to transfer important health information between providers and a date can be set for when the transition takes place. More information on health care transitions is available on the AAP National Center for Medical Home Implementation Web site and the National Health Care Transition Center Web site (www.gottransition.org).

PRIVACY AND THE ADOLESCENT EXAMINATION

As your child gets older, you may need to consider privacy during physical examinations. Properly addressing this issue during the examination of an adolescent with an autism spectrum disorder (ASD) depends greatly on the teen's developmental level. If his cognitive skills are those of a young child, it may not be appropriate for the parent to leave during the examination. In such a situation, a parent may be a source of reassurance and comfort, the same as the parent would be to a younger child with typical development who is not yet protective of his body's privacy in front of his parent.

For those adolescents—and certain preadolescents—with ASDs who are already physically modest with family or who are in the process of learning to be more modest, it is customary for the parent to step out of the room for the physical examination.

It is critically important to communicate in advance what the physical examination involves. Effective communication will help ensure that there is no misunderstanding about the reasons for and conduct of the examination.

If the patient is an adolescent or young adult and the examination requires visualizing or touching sensitive private areas, the American Academy of Pediatrics recommends a chaperone. The chaperone is usually a nurse or medical assistant rather than a friend or family member. However, using a chaperone should be a shared decision between the patient and physician. The patient's preference should be given the highest priority when deciding whether to use one.

If a medical chaperone is necessary and the patient refuses, the patient and parent should be given alternatives. These could include not performing the complete examination, performing the full examination at another time, performing it without a chaperone, or seeking care elsewhere.

SAFE TRAVELS

Parents of adults with autism spectrum disorders need to make sure that their adult children are safe travelers, whether the adult drives, rides a bike, walks, takes public transportation, or has another way of getting around the community. Even as a passenger, they must be able to self-monitor and refrain from distracting the driver and must be comfortable wearing a seat belt.

Behavioral Concerns During Adolescence

Certain psychiatric disorders such as anxiety, depression, and mood disorders may become more pronounced as your child ages. Some children may be prone to anxiety or depression, especially if they become more aware of being different from their peers. Children with greater behavioral volatility may become more unsafe as their bodies mature and develop. For example, the tantrum of a 3-year-old boy with an ASD may be no different than that of a 13-year-old boy, except that when the older boy hits it may be more injurious to himself or those around him.

If your child is struggling with difficult behaviors that are affecting her daily functioning and ability to learn, it's important to talk with your child's pediatrician. The pediatrician will consider any medical conditions, such as sleep problems or seizures, that may contribute to challenging behaviors, or psychiatric conditions. It may be helpful to involve your child's entire team when behavioral problems arise. You may talk to your child's pediatrician about coordinating with educators, therapists, psychiatrists, and other specialists to develop a plan to help your family and your child.

Budding Sexuality

While children who have ASDs will have the same body changes during puberty that other children have, they may have a harder time understanding those changes. It's important to talk about sexuality with your child, using language that he can understand. This should start well before the teenage years when differences between the sexes are explained, social skills are developed, and the importance of good personal hygiene is stressed. Talking about sexuality with any child might be uncomfortable for any parent, and it may feel especially awkward if your child has an ASD. Some parents may even think they can overlook discussions about sexuality if their child has an ASD, but every adolescent deserves to be well informed about topics like abstinence, contraception, and pregnancy. Talking about sexuality has important safety aspects as well.

Children and youth with disabilities, including ASDs, have an increased risk of being sexually abused. Some children with ASDs might be more vulnerable to sexual abuse because of dependence on others for care, less developed social skills and judgment, and difficulty defending themselves or reporting abuse. These fears lead some parents to shelter their children from social opportunities or knowledge about sex. Yet lack of education means more risk for children with ASDs and other disabilities. Studies have shown that when sexual questions are addressed openly within families, the risk of abuse is lowered. Children with ASDs can learn to protect the privacy of their own bodies if they are given the knowledge to do so.

So it is clear that frank discussions about sexuality may be even *more* important for children with ASDs because they may be less likely to learn it from their friends, movies, and other sources. Much of the information that other children pick up is subtle and indirect as opposed to clear-cut and direct, making it harder for children with ASDs to grasp. In reality, it's best that children—all children, in fact—get the information from their parents. Two important aspects to discuss are sexual safety and the social issues surrounding sex.

Sexuality education isn't just about sexual intercourse. It's about your child's body and all its impending changes, the difference between public and private, appropriate touching and boundaries, and how to prevent sexual exploitation. In reality, you began teaching your child about sexuality when you taught him to lock a public bathroom door and to change in the appropriate locker room. Over time it evolves into discussions about menstruation in girls and nocturnal emissions in boys. Eventually your conversations will turn to talk about sexual intercourse and other sexual activity. Along the way, it's also important to teach your child about touch, why some forms of touch are appropriate and others are not, and what your child can do when he is inappropriately touched.

The best time to broach these subjects is well before your child reaches puberty and should be based on what your child can understand. The same instructional tools and skills you used to teach your child about other topics can be used now to teach your child about sex and sexuality. That means you may want to use visual aids, books, and stories. It might also mean breaking down lessons into a sequence of events. Most important of all, make sure you are direct and clear in your instructions. Children with ASDs like information that is clear-cut and straightforward, not nuanced and vague. And make sure to always give your child the opportunity to ask questions and to let him know you are open to questions later on. The University of Michigan has a list of resources that can help you get started at www.med. umich.edu/yourchild/topics/disabsex.htm.

OUT IN THE WORLD

Adolescence is the time when most kids become increasingly interested in the world beyond their family and home. Peers and friendships may take on greater importance, and your child may want to explore new activities and become a greater part of the community. Eventually, your child may be interested in dating, driving, and getting a job. At the same time, some of these interests may be intimidating and frightening. Fortunately, you can help your child embrace some of these interests at her own pace along with some additional coaching from you.

Strengthening Social Skills

During the teen years, the growing significance of friendships in your child's life could lead to much turmoil. For children who have ASDs, the lack of strong social skills may be an obstacle to making and keeping friends. Like all teenagers, these deficits may become more apparent to your child at this age, and feelings of being different and lonely may become more acute, more painful. Your child may also be teased or become the target of bullies.

Helping your child develop better social skills is a lifelong process. It begins with making sure your child understands what friendship is and how friends behave toward each other. For instance, your child should understand that a friend is someone who spends time with you and treats you kindly, not someone who hangs around only when other people are not available, when she needs to borrow money, or when she needs help with homework. It also involves learning how to read body language, subtle social cues, facial expressions, and warmth, sarcasm, and hostility in another person's speech.

Fortunately, social skills appear to be something that you can teach your child. Researchers at the University of California, Los Angeles (UCLA) developed the Program for the Education and Enrichment of Relationship Skills (PEERS) for motivated teens in the seventh through 12th grades who are interested in learning ways to help them make and keep friends. It is a 14-week program that uses evidence-based interventions to help teens learn important social skills and practice these skills in sessions during real play activities such as sports and board games. Parents are taught how to help their teens make and keep friends by providing feedback to their children through social coaching during weekly socialization homework assignments.

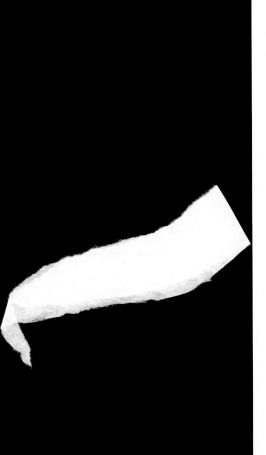

Topics in the program include how to use appropriate conversational skills, finding common interests by swapping information, using humor appropriately, and entering and exiting conversations. The program also looks at how to handle disagreements, gossip, rejection, teasing, and bullying. In addition, it looks at ways to be a good host, make phone calls, and choose the right friends. A 2009 study looking at the program found that it helped boost the social skills of children with high-functioning autism, which suggests that social skills can, in fact, be taught.

Of course, not everyone can be in the program at UCLA, but your child's pediatrician may be able to refer you to programs or classes in your area that can help. (For more information on how to access resources in your community, see Chapter 9.) You can also help your child socially by providing opportunities for her to interact with peers her age in groups and activities where she can share her interests. Encourage potential friendships by allowing your child to host get-togethers. And if your child is interested in technology, consider helping her to use appropriate social networking sites to make connections. Honor these as friendships, but teach her the right way to use this technology by sitting down with her at the computer. To find Web sites that provide discussion forums where people with autism can share their experiences, ask questions, and engage in chats, see Appendix A.

FAST FACTS: THEORY OF MIND
Theory of mind is the ability to attribute mental states—beliefs, intentions, and desires—to other people, a skill that most typical children develop and sharpen with age. Children who have autism spectrum disorders may not have well-developed theory of mind skills, making it hard for them to be empathic to other people's experiences and feelings. It is one reason why they may struggle socially. Parents can help their child develop theory of mind skills by asking what characters in books, movies, and television shows are thinking or feeling, engaging in role-play, and talking about their own thoughts and feelings.

Strengthening Community Connections

Whether we live amidst the tall skyscrapers of the city or the rural countryside of a farming town, we all live in a community, and most people need to be a part of it. Adolescence is a good time to help your child develop ways of connecting to his community. It's especially important to help your child tap into his interests and use those interests to find outlets outside the classroom.

To help your child zero in on the right activities, think about his interests. Does he love animals? Reading? Playing sports? Does he collect certain objects or play certain games? What motivates him? What are his challenges and struggles? What goals do you want to see him reach when he participates in this activity?

Some of these activities may be found in school. Most schools offer all kinds of extracurricular activities, be they sports, music programs, or chess clubs. But many of these activities can also be found in your community. The local YMCA, for instance, may offer inclusive fitness activities. Craft stores may offer classes on sewing, scrapbooking, and others arts and crafts. Churches and synagogues may have youth groups.

There are also community activities specifically for youth with ASDs. Best Buddies, an international nonprofit (www.bestbuddies.org), helps link people with ASDs to people in the community, such as corporate and civic leaders, college students, and high school students, for one-on-one friendships that can ultimately lead to employment, social opportunities, and leadership roles. Special Olympics offers the opportunity for your child to participate and compete in athletic events (www.specialolympics.org). Let your child's interests be your guide when it comes to choosing community activities.

Entering Adulthood

As a young adult, you and your child will face many decisions that will shape how she lives the rest of her life. The key is to talk about these options with your child and help her understand what she can do and what she wants to do. Like other young adults, she may be asking some important questions: "Should I go to college?" "What should I study?" "Where will I work?" Helping your child answer these questions is an important job for parents. Knowing your options will help.

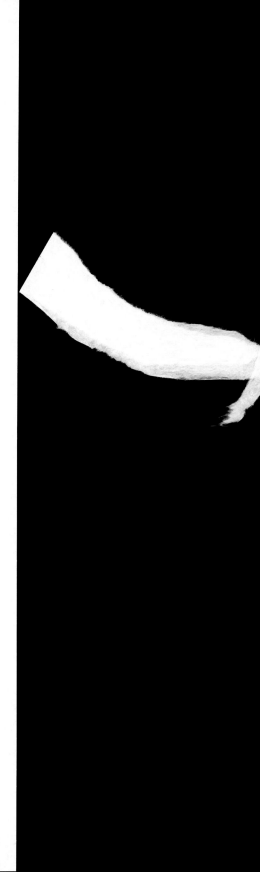

Education After High School

Not all people with ASDs want to stop attending school after they graduate high school. Some will want to pursue higher education, be it at a college, a community college, or a vocational school. Many 4-year universities and community colleges are now offering more support services for students with ASDs.

There are 3 main kinds of postsecondary education models for young adults with disabilities. In the *mixed/hybrid model,* students are in classes, for credit or audit, with students who do not have disabilities but also take life-skill classes with other students who have

---

LINGERING QUESTIONS

My son has become interested in dating. Is this possible for a boy with autism?

Yes it is. Some children with autism spectrum disorders (ASDs) will not have an interest in dating, but others, like your son, do become interested in pursuing a relationship. Unlike other activities your child will want to pursue, it will be hard for you as the parent to control your child's romantic interests and whether the feelings are reciprocated. What you can do is help your child learn basic social skills such as what to say when you want to ask someone out, how to behave, and what's appropriate. Like most people, your child may learn the sorrows of heartbreak and the joys of falling in love.

Can a teenager with an ASD drive?

It depends on your child. Some teens—typically developing and with ASDs—are not ready to be safe drivers and should wait until they are older before getting a driver's license. Gauge your child's ability to focus, coordinate his motor skills, and understand what other drivers and vehicles are doing. If you're not sure, talk to your child's pediatrician, therapists, teachers, and others involved in his care for their input. There may be specialized providers in the field of occupational therapy within your community who offer formal driving evaluations.

Where will my teenager live?

Adults with ASDs have several housing options. Some may wind up living completely independently, while others may live in supported living, supervised living, or group homes, each with varying degrees of supervision, assistance, and support. In choosing where your child will live, consider his safety skills, phone skills, and ability to maintain and clean a home. Other important skills include grocery shopping, cooking, budgeting, and doing laundry.

disabilities. Students also get work experience on or off campus. In the *substantially separate model,* students participate solely in classes with other students who have disabilities. They may participate in social activities on campus and may acquire some work experience on or off campus. In the *inclusive individual support model,* students get individualized services such as an educational coach, tutor, or technology in college courses, certificate programs, or degree programs, for audit or credit. Services and employment experiences are driven by the student's career goals.

Preparing the transition plan can help your child zero in on her interests and goals. It's also important to have regular discussions about his future plans. Don't hesitate to consult experts such as your child's pediatrician, a school guidance counselor, college admissions professionals, and even parents of older children.

Job Options

Like most people, young adults with ASDs may someday seek employment. Some may first attend community college or college, but others may go directly into the workforce. The desire to be trained in a skill or profession and become gainfully employed is a major transition, one that shapes a lot of your child's future.

Transition planning in the IEP was designed to get you and your child to start thinking about possible job directions. One of the best things your child can do is to explore job options while still in middle and high school. Learning about career opportunities that exist, participating in school-to-work activities such as internships, and identifying specific areas of interest will help your child prepare for a job and get the training she might need if she has skill deficits. Your county or school district may provide vocational rehabilitation (VR) or planning services. (See "Vocational Rehabilitation" on the next page.) Your child may even be able to get some work experiences right in school by helping with light office duties, staffing the school store, or assisting in the cafeteria. Your school may even have formalized programs that support these types of job experiences, which you should explore. Outside school, your child may be able to secure a paid or unpaid internship.

People with ASDs and other disabilities may have different work environments that vary in several ways. The job setting your child chooses will depend on the extent of her abilities and interests. Some adults with ASDs, for instance, may work in competitive employment, with market wages, typical job responsibilities, and no long-term support. Some may benefit from working in supported employment, which offers competitive employment but with support services on the job. Another option is secured or segregated employment, in which individuals with disabilities work separately from workers without disabilities and do tasks such as sorting, assembling, and collating. Sheltered employment is similar in that workers are segregated, but this type of work provides training and services that help workers develop life skills.

Vocational Rehabilitation

In addition to protecting people with disabilities from discrimination, the federal Rehabilitation Act offers VR, a program that funds training and education so that a person with disabilities may secure a job. Vocational rehabilitation programs are managed by individual states and funded largely by the federal government.

To be eligible, you must have a physical or mental impairment that may limit your ability to secure a job and show that you require VR services to become employed. You must also prove that you intend to work.

To participate in a VR program, your child must first submit an application. Once the application is approved, your child will complete an Individualized Plan for Employment (IPE). The IPE outlines goals and the services offered to meet those goals. Vocational rehabilitation offers a range of services including career counseling, skills assessments, job training, and assistive technology. Services end, or are closed out, after you have been at your job for at least 90 days. The services may also be discontinued if it appears the goal of securing a job cannot be met or if the individual chooses to drop out of the program.

In recent years, growing numbers of people with ASDs have been accessing VR services, according to a report by the Institute for Community Inclusion. In fact, the number of young adults with ASDs who closed out of VR more than tripled between 2003 and 2008. The study found that young adults with ASDs were more likely than those with intellectual or other disabilities to receive assessment, job placement, and on-the-job support. Those who received these services were also more likely to get a job.

Down the Road

Perhaps the most critical—and often most frightening—question that parents face is, "Who will take care of my child someday when I am no longer around?" Some adults with ASDs will be able to hold down a job, live independently, and even have a family. Others will be able to do so with supports and assistance. Still others, however, will benefit from living in residential facilities that offer more support, such as group homes.

Planning for your child's future often involves meeting with attorneys, financial planners, and others who can help you work out the specific details. If you think your child will require long-term care and living arrangements, you should start making plans before he turns 18 and is legally an adult. If, at age 18 years, your young adult is not able to make responsible decisions, a formal evaluation should be done to determine if he needs a legal guardian. Guardianship is not an easy issue, especially if your adult child has difficulty with problem-solving skills in some areas but can make some decisions on his own in others. Guardianship means that other people will help your child make decisions about his health and other aspects of his life. So it should be pursued only when you are sure that your child is unable to make well-thought-out decisions for himself about health care choices as well as choices related to daily life and finances. You may want to talk to your child's pediatrician, service coordinator, school team, and immediate family members about this decision. An attorney may also be helpful. For more information, search for guardianship at the National Health Care Transition Center (www.gottransition.org).

It's also important to make sure your adult child receives adequate health care coverage and is financially secure. Establishing a special needs trust can help do this (see "Special Needs Trust" on page 201 in Chapter 10).

Accessing appropriate resources in your community is necessary to help pave the way for a smooth transition from adolescence through the teen years and into adulthood. By working with your transition team to create a plan well ahead of any major changes, you will help ensure that your child has the skills and supports he will need to feel successful and fulfilled during his adult life.

Autism Champion: Tim Page

Tim Page had always been passionate about music, even at the tender age of 2 when a song could ease an unruly tantrum. As a child, he played piano and composed music. He went on to become a Pulitzer Prize-winning music critic for *The Washington Post*. But his childhood was fraught with challenges. "I flunked almost everything," Tim recalls. "I was still peeing my pants when I was 12. I was unable to concentrate in class. I couldn't understand why teachers would want me to do this or do that. I was incredibly awkward and couldn't play any sports."

Tim grew up in the 1950s and early 1960s, when autism was less recognized and poorly understood. He hated being made to learn things that didn't interest him and always preferred it when people explained why they did what they did. His father insisted he make eye contact. But it was difficult for him to give or receive hugs and touches from anybody outside his family, a deficit that had it been corrected, he says, would have made a big difference in almost every aspect of his life.

Reading *Emily Post's Etiquette* helped him understand social nuances and why people behaved the way they did. When he was finally diagnosed with Asperger syndrome at 45, everything made sense. His experience became his memoir, *Parallel Play*.

Today, the 56-year-old divorced father of 3 sons—one of whom has Asperger syndrome—is a journalism and music professor at the University of Southern California. He talks openly about his experience with Asperger syndrome and says children with Asperger syndrome are better off when they're left to pursue their own interests, which for Page was music, old records, and silent films.

As an adult, he says he has mastered the art of "playing Tim Page" and can speak to large audiences with ease. But he still struggles with social situations where he doesn't know anyone, rarely attends social outings with his colleagues, and generally prefers his own company to that of others. He continues to dread any form of overstimulation, be it loud noises, busy conversations, colors, or lights, and struggles with eye contact when discussing anything he feels deeply about or listening to music with others.

"What I've done is find ways I can be at my best and not at my worst," Tim says. "I know what I can do easily, and if I have to do something that is more difficult, I find a way of talking myself into it. These days, I usually come through."

CHAPTER 12

Putting It All Together: Everyday Strategies for Helping Your Child

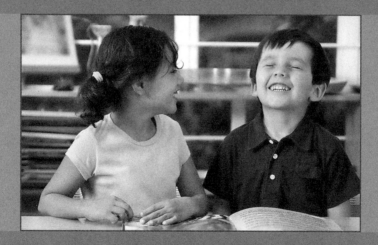

Imagine if you could anticipate your child's every move, every day. You'd know exactly what would upset him in any situation. You'd know his every mood and anticipate all his needs. You'd know exactly what to expect at any social gathering, public event, and outing. And you'd have a strategy on hand for dealing with every problem that arises.

Of course, as you know, real life doesn't work that way, especially where children are involved. Like anyone, your child with an autism spectrum disorder (ASD) is full of surprises, good and bad, and you just never know what will happen on any given day. It's important that you accept that fact right from the start, which will make unexpected and unwanted behaviors less daunting.

Then you need to come up with a collection of strategies for coping with different situations. Keep in mind that even if you do find something that works, you have to realize that what works for your child in one situation may not continue to be effective at another point in time. It's important that you are prepared with plan B—and while you're at it, thinking about plans C, D, and E. Remember that problem solving requires being creative, flexible, and patient.

Dealing successfully with whatever the challenge might be involves being prepared for the unexpected. It's also about knowing that there are multiple ways to tackle any problem. There is usually no single universally correct solution for most challenges faced by parents of children with ASDs.

In this chapter, we'll provide some practical strategies for parents on how to help their child with an ASD navigate the world. We can't possibly identify every situation and provide solutions for each one. But we hope these personal stories will help you come up with your own strategies and ideas. The key is to think creatively and find a solution that works for you and your child at any given moment.

Getting Through the Day

All of us have routines and schedules that we must follow, even children. When children have problems with their routines, it can be difficult for you as the parent to get through your day. Simple tasks like getting dressed, eating a snack, or getting in the car can become a monumental challenge, and you wind up feeling stressed and exhausted.

Most parents who have children with ASDs have come up with ways to deal with these difficult moments. In this section, we'll hear from these parents and learn how they have managed.

A Penchant for Routine

"Like most children with autism, my 4-year old son Quennedy likes predictability. When he came home from school, he used to run and run. He was filled with anxiety.

"So when I saw him at school using a visual schedule, I decided to try this at home. We drew up a schedule with pictures of washing hands, going potty, eating snack, and reading a book. Then, we'd end every evening with a short movie or video.

"Having this visual schedule calmed him right down. If he wants to know what's next, all he has to do is look at the schedule. If there are unexpected activities like a dentist visit, I make a new visual icon and show him the picture. So when we took him to his first dental visit, I drew a stick figure and a chair, and showed him what was coming. It didn't work great the first time. But he was much better on his second visit."—Tracey, Cincinnati, OH

Being on Time

"When Terry is late, he gets very anxious. It used to cause serious meltdowns. Over the years—he's 14 now—I've learned to make sure we leave super early for anything Terry does and that we build plenty of travel time into our plans when we go to movies, appointments, dinner dates, and other outings.

"We recently went to see a play and had to leave directly from church. My husband and I both knew we'd get there in plenty of time. But Terry was anxious the whole way there. Every red light, every slow car, and my husband's wrong turn all ratcheted up his anxiety. By the time we got there he was so tense. To make matters worse, we had to deal with very tight crowds, and our seats were in the middle of the row. Everyone was chattering, and the whole event turned into a real struggle for him.

"My second adaptation, I decided, needs to be getting aisle seats for these kinds of events so he can get up and move without disturbing people and he doesn't feel claustrophobic."
—Delia, Voorheesville, NY

Brushing Teeth

"My daughter Annie, who is now 9, always hated to brush her teeth. She didn't like the way it felt, didn't have the patience to sit still for me while I did it, and was terrified of going to the dentist. To help with brushing and dental visits, we started counting very slowly—so I have enough time to brush—from 1 to 5 on the bottom teeth and 6 through 10 on the top. When I get to 5, she repeats it, and then I move on to 6.

"Counting gives her predictability, an end in sight, and she has to participate, or I keep brushing until she makes an attempt to communicate. Counting, in general, soothes her. Singing songs like ABCs, 'Itsy Bitsy Spider,' and 'Five Little Ducks' has also been helpful for her."—Amy, Exton, PA

Tying His Shoes

"When my son was young—he's now 34—he insisted on tying his own shoes. The laces always wound up loose and large. He didn't like the laces to touch the floor, so he constantly stopped to retie them, often in midstream where people would run into him.

"This didn't work because he couldn't tie them tight enough. We decided to permanently tie them with a double knot. We made the laces loose enough so he could slide his foot in and out of the shoe easily but tight enough so the shoe wouldn't come off his foot."
—Phyllis, Kansas City, KS

Being Away From Home

"Traveling, particularly overnights, can be very trying on kids with autism. If there was a sink in the same room, Annie always wanted to play with water. To solve this, we put her in a 5-man tent in the room and called it 'Annie's own tent.' We also put a blow-up air mattress in it. She loves it. She knows it's her own space, and she feels very safe being enclosed in it.

"I also bring a plastic container with her favorite toys in it, so she has her own play box, and her special blanket or whatever stuffed animal she likes at the time. Then we fasten the zipper and tie a bow around the 2 zippers so she can't get out. In order to watch her, we invested in a video monitor that we angled at the tent, so we could hear and watch everything Annie did. This has proven to be a very effective way to make a safe environment for Annie and allow me to sleep."—Amy, Exton, PA

Driving Different Routes

"My son Sam loves routine, like most children on the spectrum. Whenever we break from routine, he gets very anxious. He used to get anxious if I took a different route to get somewhere. To break him of that, I'd deliberately take a different route and then give him a reward. He came to associate changes in routes with getting a reward."—Barbara, Ann Arbor, MI

Teaching Him to Get Dressed

"Our son CJ is 4 and learning how to dress himself. To teach him, we created a visual schedule that outlines the order of what he puts on—underwear, socks, shirt, and pants.

"He starts by looking at the schedule and then walks over and retrieves the first item. Then he looks at the second item and gets that. And so on. Sometimes, it takes a long time for him to get dressed, but he is learning how to do it. It just has to be at his own pace."
—Ronny, Cincinnati, OH

Helping Her Identify Herself

"Because Annie is nonverbal, she couldn't tell someone where she lives if she is lost. So we have a medical bracelet (made of stainless steel) that is permanently on her left wrist. I snuck it on her wrist one night when she was 2 and asleep. She just woke up with it and couldn't get it off.

"The bracelet says her full name and identifies her as 'nonverbal, autism.' It also has her address and my cell phone number. We taught her to point at the bracelet when someone asks her, 'What's your name?' That way she can interact with them and knows where the information is should she need to tell someone."—Amy, Exton, PA

Afraid of Transitions

"For the longest time, our son would have a fit every time we went on a walk and turned around to come home. We had no idea what was making him so upset. He even hated it if I had to turn the car around in the driveway and go back the way I came. His tantrums could go on long after we came home. Finally, one day, he said, 'Other way.' That's when we figured it out.

"He wasn't being bratty or a baby. He was really scared. I offered to hold his hand or carry him. He wanted to be held. Now we know to announce that we are turning around before we do. By acknowledging his tantrum and then comforting him, he was able to calm down and go on. We make several announcements now with every transition from having dinner to getting a bath."—Ronny, Cincinnati, OH

Tap Into Technology

"We bought an iPad, and my daughter Rory took it over. She loves it! It has become a major teaching tool. We have gotten a lot of apps for her and most them aren't so-called 'autism apps.'

"One that has really helped is called *Shape Builder,* where you can see the outlines of shapes and drag shapes over into a puzzle. I am convinced this is why she is now writing. She had very poor fine motor skills, and they are significantly improved. *ABC Tracer* is another app good for learning to write letters.

"She also loves *Kid Calculator* and has learned a lot about numbers. She can identify numbers up to 100. She uses a drawing app called *Starfall ABCs* to write words. She also likes the flash card apps and has had fun pronouncing all the different kinds of dog breeds, car types, and lots of other categories. They are called *Baby Flash Cards*. There are also *ABA Flash Cards* and ABA receptive card apps. Rory has absorbed so much from the different apps, gained motor strength, and figured things out on her own. It's incredible."—Nora, Gaithersburg, MD

🐾 🐾 🐾 🐾 🐾

You may find some of these ideas helpful and some not as helpful. Whatever you try, don't get frustrated too quickly or give up too soon. Change can be met with resistance, and you and your child are making a change together. So you may need to try something new several times before you get a positive response, or give a highly desired item or activity to reward the behavior. You may also want to make sure that other people in your home are helping you make this change and that you and your partner are on the same page and both agree to try the change.

Dealing With Maladaptive Behaviors

Maladaptive behaviors are those behaviors that are inappropriate, disruptive, and not beneficial. In children who have ASDs, they may be behaviors that are stereotypic, ritualistic, self-injurious, or aggressive. Sometimes they may be tantrums. In a classroom, your child may run around the room, talk loudly, or disrupt the lesson. It's important to note that although these behaviors can appear "bad" to you, they may be serving an important function for your child.

Most children with ASDs who engage in maladaptive behaviors do so when they are anxious, afraid, or confused. Many don't know how to communicate effectively, so they resort to behaviors that are counterproductive and often downright annoying. The problem is, these behaviors may interfere with your child's ability to learn and may make it difficult to participate in group settings.

Putting an end to maladaptive behaviors isn't easily done, but limiting your child's outbursts can be done, especially if you know the function of your child's behavior. As we have said, many children with ASDs become anxious when routines change without warning, or when they are in an unfamiliar situation or frustrated with a new task. Parents can help lessen maladaptive behaviors by trying to reduce their child's anxiety whenever possible. Here are some ways to do that.

- *Be clear and precise when you speak to your child about the behavior you expect from her.* Children with ASDs can't "read between the lines" and have a hard time discerning facial expressions. When communicating with your child, always say what you mean and mean what you say. Avoid the use of metaphors, idioms, and sarcasm to make your point.
- *Give any direction in simple one-step sentences.* Allow up to 30 seconds (sometimes longer) for your child to take in your verbal direction, process it, formulate a response, and respond. This may feel like a long time, but children with ASDs process and respond slower than a typically developing child.
- *Give your child time to do what needs to be done.* It often takes children with ASDs longer to complete a task, so patience is critical. If you know your child needs more time, build it into the task. This means adding "get ready" time to your schedule when you are leaving to go somewhere or transitioning from one activity to the next. Some parents find it helpful to set a kitchen or microwave timer to help with time management.
- *Be consistent with your response.* For example, if tantrums occur, it is important that your response be consistent. This way your child will not be confused about what is appropriate.
- *Use positive reinforcement.* Give your child a reason to behave appropriately, not just a reason to avoid an undesirable behavior.
- *Remember to tell your child what she did right, not just what she did wrong.*
- *Stay on a predictable schedule as much as possible.* Children with ASDs often become highly anxious when routines change unexpectedly. Let your child know if something out of the ordinary is happening that day. You can do this verbally or by using visual cards or telling a social story.

- *Remain as calm as you can.* It is understandable that it can be hard to remain cool and collected during stressful situations. One suggestion is to use a gentle tone of voice, presenting facts without any emotion, and providing information in a logical sequence.
- *Use a visual schedule as much as possible.* Many classrooms use one. This is because children with ASDs are generally visual learners, rather than auditory (verbal) learners. Some parents also find it helpful to ask a teacher or therapist to make a visual schedule, especially if they do not have a computer or printer.

Before the Behavior Begins

Of course, it helps if you can anticipate and prevent maladaptive behaviors. That's why it's important to be on the lookout for what Brenda Smith Myles, PhD, calls the *rage cycle*. According to Dr Myles, an expert on autism, rage occurs for a reason and typically runs through 3 stages: rumbling, meltdown/rage, and recovery.

Common behaviors during the rumbling stage, which occurs before your child has a complete tantrum or meltdown, include biting of the nails or lips, lowering the voice, tensing muscles, tapping the foot, grimacing, and other indications of discontent. Here are some ways to stop the meltdown in the rumbling stage. Keep in mind they may be used at home or in the classroom.

- *Use gentle touch.* Assume a child is tapping his foot loudly. By gently touching his leg or foot, he may stop the behavior.
- *Show interest in your child's interests.* If your child doesn't want to do the task before him, tell him you know he prefers doing something else. By acknowledging his interests, you may deflect inappropriate behavior.
- *Take your child on a walk.* Allow him to break away from the situation and go on a walk with him instead. While you're walking, let your child say what's on his mind without punishment.
- *Remove your child from the situation completely.* Send him on an errand such as getting something from his bedroom, fetching the mail, or dropping off something at a neighbor's.

- *Send the child to a safe place where he can regain his composure.*
- *Be sensitive to your child's sensory issues.* Whether it's loud noises, noxious smells, or strange textures, many children with ASDs have strong preferences or dislikes for certain things that affect their senses. Try to figure out which ones your child likes, and accommodate those. For instance, if he doesn't like hugs, don't insist that he accept one from an adoring relative. If he dislikes loud noises, avoid driving past the fire station. If he's sensitive to smells, skip the perfumed shampoos, soaps, and lotions.
- *Give your child a saying he can use in difficult moments.* You might suggest he repeat the phrase, "This will go away," or "Take a deep breath."
- *Look your child in the eye when reaffirming a rule that has been broken.* Avoid engaging in long discussions about who's right and who's wrong. Simply tell him what's expected of him, and move on.
- *Analyze meltdowns.* Consider what was happening in the hours before your child began showing problem behaviors, and try to avoid similar circumstances in the future. Come up with strategies to help yourself stay calm during an episode. Devise ways that you can try to soothe your child next time. Doing an antecedent, behavior, consequence observation form, as discussed in Chapter 5, can help too.
- *Try a little humor.* Whether it's deflecting your child's anxiety or taming the irate glare of an onlooker, a funny comment can sometimes turn the situation into a laughable moment. Make sure your child understands the humor, however, so he doesn't think you're making fun of him. With onlookers, it can help to simply say something like, "I guess he's having a bad day."

For information on the complete rage cycle and other helpful strategies, see Chapter 5, pages 111 through 114.

WHAT ARE SOCIAL STORIES?

Social stories help improve a child's understanding of certain events while teaching appropriate social skills and behaviors. They often take the form of a storybook that you make about a challenging activity for your child (like getting a haircut). Sentences may be factual, descriptive, or affirmative, or they may acknowledge a feeling or opinion by the writer or others. The situation is described in detail and focuses on important social cues, events, and reactions your child might expect to occur in the situation. They may also include the actions and reactions that might be expected of your child, and why. For examples, see The Gray Center Web site at www.thegraycenter.org.

Encourage Your Child's Social Skills

Most children—and adults too—take their social skills for granted. Early on, they learn how to enter a playgroup and join in with other children. Over time, they learn to read body language and facial expressions and can sense when someone is losing interest in the topic of conversation. They also learn how to safely leave an interaction without offending the other person. For a child who has an ASD, such basic social skills can be a challenge and may seem like impossible tasks. Many children with ASDs may have difficulty engaging in one-on-one interactions, reading body language, and initiating play. Often, they struggle with empathy and have trouble understanding the emotions of others.

For children with ASDs, social skills need to be taught, explicitly and regularly. It's important to know that just because a child doesn't interact with her peers doesn't mean the desire isn't there. She may simply lack the skills that allow for social engagement. Here are some ways that you can help your child develop and hone those skills.

- *Play games that teach social skills, body language, and facial expressions.* Games like charades may be especially effective. Or you can try watching a TV show with the volume turned off. Pause the show and ask your child what the person is feeling and might say. Then turn the volume back on and play the show. See if your child is correct.
- *Provide direct instructions on what your child could say or do.* Children with ASDs need clear information. While demonstrating specific skills, state out loud what she could do and say in different situations.

- *Mind-reading games can be used to teach children with ASDs to understand the perspective of others.* Looking at pictures of various situations, a child is asked to describe the thoughts and feelings of the people in the picture.

- *Watch movies and TV shows for teaching facial expressions, body language, and good manners.* Encourage your child to pay attention to how emotions are revealed in these expressions. Talk about what the expressions mean, so your child can better understand how others are feeling or thinking.

- *Act out difficult social interactions.* Start by role-playing situations using scripts. As your child's skills improve, let your child improvise what she would say or do.

- *Use social stories to teach your child how to socialize.*

- *Let your child spend time with typically developing peers.*

- *Enlist teachers, teaching assistants, and recess aides in helping to promote your child's social skills.* Ask the teacher to pair up your child with a classroom "buddy" who shares your child's interests. Ask a recess aide to find a child who can interact with your child when they're on the playground. Suggest that teachers and teaching assistants create group activities that give your child the chance to display her special talents.

- *Teach your child conversational listening skills.* Children with ASDs may be listening to someone but not understand why it's important to let that other person know that she's listening. Encourage your child to nod her head or make an acknowledging comment as simple as "Wow!" or "Really?"

- *Look for ways to get your child involved in extracurricular activities.* Whether it's sports, a club, or a group focused on a specific hobby or interest, the key is exposing your child to a wide range of opportunities to build friendships and have social interactions. It is important to note, though, that a child with an ASD in an extracurricular sport may need some extra support. Team sports may be more demanding and harder to navigate socially. If your child needs this extra support, your local parks and recreation department may offer adaptive recreational activities that your child will enjoy. Some families find that individual sports (for example, swimming, martial arts, running) foster their child's self-esteem and make recreation more accessible. They main thing is, choose something that is fun for your child!

My child has trouble finding solutions to simple problems.
What can I do to help?

Try narrating your actions to him, or *living out loud,* as Brenda Smith Myles, PhD, calls it. Living out loud helps your child better understand his environment and what he can do when he's confronted with a problem. For instance, let's say you lock your keys in the car. You might want to say, "I'm going to stay calm. Now I will call Daddy at work. He's not there. I will call our neighbor Mrs Smith, who has a key. She is home. She will bring me the key." Narrating your actions teaches your child the step-by-step process of solving a problem and reassures him that most problems can be managed without a meltdown.

When Your Child Goes to School

Once your child enters school, his daily routine is no longer entirely in your hands. At this point, it becomes important to communicate your child's unique needs to teachers, administrators, therapists, and support staff at school. Some people may know very little about ASDs, while others may be highly skilled and trained to work with children who have ASDs. As the parent, you can help teachers better understand what will help them teach your child. Here are some things you can do.

- *Ask about creating a visual schedule.* Children with ASDs like predictability, and being able to see what's in store for them can make life at school less stressful. But always remind your child that changes can and will occur, so that he is not completely caught off guard by the unexpected fire drill or special event.
- *Teach your child to listen for instructions for other children.* If a teacher tells one student to stop talking, it's a good idea for your child to stay quiet too.
- *Ask the teacher to organize a circle of friends for your child.* Being accepted by peers is important to school-aged children. Ask the teacher if there are students who might make good buddies for your child. These students should be socially astute and open to allowing your child to spend time with them.
- *Share your child's interests with his teachers.* Knowing what your child likes will allow teachers to use that topic when they want to engage your child while delivering a lesson.

- *Ask the teacher to provide your child with a safe space or cooling-off area.* A space in the classroom, such as a table or special chair, may be tried first. If unsuccessful, a calming area outside the classroom, perhaps an office, should be designated. The idea is to give your child a place to go when he becomes overwhelmed and needs to calm down.
- *Find out if your child can have some downtime during the day.* Spending a day at school can be stressful for some children. Giving them the opportunity to relax can be reassuring to them and make new activities less stressful.
- *Encourage teachers to be specific and precise when giving instructions.* Children with ASDs need clear instructions about what to do and what's expected of them. Simply telling them to clean their desks is often not enough. It's important to tell them exactly what that means. To be clearer, it's better to ask students to put away their notebooks.
- *Praise often.* A simple compliment stated simply, clearly, and specifically can make a world of difference for a child who has an ASD and can give him the confidence he needs to do well. Urge your child's teachers to find moments when your child has done something well and to point those out to him.
- *Break down tasks into smaller components.* Give students a step-by-step description of each mini-task that needs to be done to complete an assignment.
- *Make yourself available to the teacher.* Don't just outline a list of demands. Offer to assist the teacher with understanding your child and provide strategies for dealing with problems. Be patient and realize that not all teachers will know how to handle a student with an ASD.
- *Reinforce school activities at home.* At home, try using some of the teacher's tools, such as a Picture Exchange Communication System book, visual schedule, or math manipulatives like pattern blocks or interlocking cubes. This can help your child be less anxious in class and generalize the skills he is learning at school.

Taking Care of You

You might wonder why a chapter on helping your child has a section about helping you, the child's primary caregiver. It's the classic "oxygen mask" scenario. When you're on an airplane, you're always told to put the oxygen mask on yourself first before you put it on your child. Only by helping yourself are you better able to take care of your child—any child, for that matter.

- *Keep a list of friends and professional resources you can call to discuss problems.* Enlist their help for practical assistance if you need it.
- *Exercise regularly.* Regular activity releases stress, helps you sleep, and improves your mood. Make time to hit the gym, take a walk, or do some gentle stretching. Do it with a friend and you'll build in some social time too.
- *Consider joining a support group.* Spending time with others who are on the same journey you are can lessen your stress, give you new coping strategies, and provide you with much-needed information.
- *Find ways to reduce stress.* Whether it's a monthly massage or a weekly lunch with a friend, look for ways to lower your stress. Raising a child who has an ASD can be extremely stressful. Taking time to rest and rejuvenate can help you be a better parent.
- *Try to get your own sleep.* Easier said than done, perhaps, but a good night's rest can give you the stamina it takes to raise all children. Make sleep a priority in your schedule.

Autism Champion: Carrie Mason-Sears, PhD

As a clinical child psychologist, Carrie Mason-Sears, PhD, says working with children who have ASDs is a lot like solving a mystery. "It's finding out how a child thinks and encodes emotions," she says. "That's the fun part for me."

Once she rules out any physical conditions causing their behavioral problems, she sets out to find a way to work with a child using strategies and devices that the child can understand. "It's all about trying to engage them in a way that's meaningful to them," says Dr Mason-Sears, who is in private practice in Cincinnati, OH. "Once you speak their language, you can give them a tool to manage their behavior."

Dr Mason-Sears recently created a Stump Monster to help a little girl who got "stumped" and threw tantrums whenever she was asked to do something she wasn't sure she could handle. The Stump Monster was a character the girl could tame. "We could ward it off, trap it, or ask him a clarifying question," Dr Mason-Sears says.

Years ago, she worked with a boy who paced and did rhythmic movements whenever he was anxious. Because the boy liked water and hydraulic systems, Dr Mason-Sears created a thermostat to help him define his emotions. If the thermostat was blue, it meant he was calm. When he felt anger coming on, he entered the orange phase. Red, and he was in a full-blown rage. "For children with autism, emotions are very vague," Dr Mason-Sears recalls. "It's hard for them to define what mad is. If you can find a metaphor with something the child understands—like water systems and color coding—then they have a way to describe it that they understand."

Dr Mason-Sears got her start as an intern at the Treatment and Education of Autistic and Related Communication-Handicapped Children (TEACCH) Center at the University of North Carolina in Chapel Hill. Since she started her career in 1994, she says she's worked with hundreds of children with ASDs.

"The number one thing parents should do is to connect with their child on something that has meaning to the child," she says. "If they like Pokémon, then learn about Pokémon. If they line up cars, line up cars. If they perseverate, get in their way and get them to notice you. The key is to create some kind of meaningful connection, and that becomes the foundation for everything."

CHAPTER 13

Autism Spectrum Disorders and Our Family

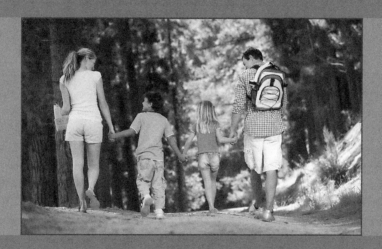

Asher's mother, Carly, loves her son and celebrates his accomplishments, no matter how small. But accepting his diagnosis of autism and adjusting to the changes that Asher brings to her and her family has been a journey. As you will see, she has made sacrifices and adjustments to accommodate Asher's disability, but the joys that her children bring are worth it. Before Asher, she had what she considered an idyllic life. After Asher, she still has a great life. On some levels her dreams have changed, but her journey has taught her that new dreams can be just as sweet.

Right from the start, Asher, who is now 7 years old, presented his family with several challenges. He was a "runner" who, without close supervision, could disappear from the house. Because of his sensory needs, he sometimes played rough with his sisters, broke their toys, and jumped on their beds. Perhaps the biggest obstacle was his difficulty communicating his wants and needs. As any mother would, Carly worked tirelessly to help her son communicate more effectively. She researched strategies to make sure she was using good methods. All the while she worried—about Asher and his future, about his younger sister who was at higher risk for developing an autism spectrum disorder (ASD), and about how all of this would affect her family. All the stress began to take its toll, and Carly began showing signs of depression and anxiety. Luckily, through the support of her family and community, she is doing better.

Asher's autism has affected everyone in the family. Carly and her husband do their best to work as a team, but like all parents, she sometimes takes out her frustrations on her spouse. Asher's younger sister has trouble understanding why Asher can leave the dinner table without eating all his food but she can't. Asher's disability sometimes means that going out as a family to a restaurant or traveling for a vacation can present unique challenges and has at times led the family to feel isolated.

Still, Carly has worked hard to include Asher in as much as he can do. She has encouraged her daughters to do the same. "Because he doesn't talk, they forget that he can be talked to," Carly says. Even though there are times when she gets discouraged, she continues to support Asher by making the adjustments he needs to be successful. They've fenced in the yard, installed the proper locks, and adjusted their expectations. "You just learn to celebrate the small things," she says. "With my girls, it might be winning a race. With Asher, it's when he learns to use a fork."

As this story demonstrates, the diagnosis of an ASD can have a tremendous effect on a family. It can cause stress on a marriage and create turmoil for siblings. It can limit activities and social outings. It can burden finances and employment opportunities. For mothers, who are frequently the primary caregiver, caring for a child with an ASD may even result in mental health issues.

At the same time, families say having a child with autism can bring unspeakable joy and incredible rewards. Small milestones that may go unnoticed in children with typical development are celebrated at every turn in children who have ASDs. And many parents speak of the deep appreciation they feel for their child.

Just as every child with an ASD is different, so too is every family. While all families go through stressful times, studies have shown that families of children who have ASDs often experience higher levels of stress than families who do not. In this chapter, we'll look at the effect of ASDs on loved ones, what families can do to buffer themselves from stressors, and ways everyone in the family can embrace this new challenge, even gaining strength from the experience.

How Autism Spectrum Disorders Affect Marriages

The effect of ASDs on your relationship with your spouse is as varied as marriages themselves. Some couples come together and share the dream of raising a child who attains his full potential. Others become divided in how to raise the child, and one partner may even deny the diagnosis. Still others may struggle but remain committed to keeping their partnership together. Like any union, whether a marriage affected by ASDs survives depends on numerous factors.

For years, people thought that many marriages involving a child with an ASD ended in divorce. But a study released in 2010 by researchers at the Kennedy Krieger Institute found that 64% of children with an ASD remain with both parents, a percentage that is no different than for children without an ASD.

FAMILY MATTERS

My husband doesn't provide much help when it comes to caring for our son. How do I get him more involved?

It's not unusual for one parent—often the mother—to become the lead caregiver for a child with an autism spectrum disorder (ASD). Men tend to have a more difficult time dealing with situations that do not have a straightforward solution and may instead put their energies into other things. In reality, however, both parents should be sharing in the day-to-day responsibilities. Let your husband know how you would value his participation and specific ways he can help. If he is trying, make sure you are thankful even if he is helping in a different way than you would have. You might also suggest he talk to a therapist if he's having trouble accepting the diagnosis. Invite him to your child's appointments so that he can learn more about ASDs and how he can be more involved. Some fathers may struggle learning how to connect with children with ASDs, so you might try to find an activity just for them that will help them create a stronger bond.

My husband and I want to go out once in a while, but we worry about finding a babysitter who can manage our daughter with autism. Where can we look for sitters?

Try looking for someone in the National Respite Network at http://archrespite.org/home. You might find babysitters through a local college or university, especially if it has a special education program. Summer camp counselors who care for children with ASDs make great babysitters during the school year. You might also find help through Family Voices (www.familyvoices.org) or the National Center for Family/Professional Partnerships (www.fv-ncfpp.org). If you belong to a church or synagogue, you may find help from fellow members. Local chapters of autism organizations may help you locate a sitter too.

My grandson was just diagnosed with autism. What does this mean for me as the grandparent?

For most grandparents, having a grandchild with an ASD means having another grandchild to love and cherish. But a recent survey found that having a grandchild with an ASD can have a profound effect on grandparents and may shape where they live and how they spend their retirement savings. Some grandparents move to be near their grandchild with autism, while others contribute money to treatments. An amazing 70% even become involved with treatment decisions. Not surprisingly, many worry a great deal about their adult children and the stressors they face. Like parents, grandparents may want to learn as much as they can about ASDs. Understanding ASDs can help you become a more effective and compassionate grandparent.

Another study done at the University of Wisconsin-Madison Waisman Center was less optimistic; that study found that parents of grown children with autism were more likely to divorce than couples whose children did not have autism. So while the divorce rate between the 2 groups of parents was the same when the child was younger than 8 years, the rate went up after that for parents of children with an ASD and down for parents of children without disabilities. According to the study, the prolonged needs of a child with an ASD last longer for these couples, causing greater strain on the marriage. The study found that the rate of divorce was higher in moms who were younger at the time they gave birth to the child with an ASD and when the child with an ASD was born later in the birth order. Other studies have linked higher rates of divorce in families with a child with other disabilities, such as attention-deficit/hyperactivity disorder.

Despite these findings, experts say that the key to a good marriage involving a child with an ASD is the same as it is for other marriages: communicating honestly and openly, spending time together, and providing support to one another. Studies have found that mothers in particular stress the importance of spousal support, of having a partner who knows the routine, and splitting the responsibilities. Working together, being flexible, and having someone who is willing to share feelings and concerns is also important.

Challenges for Siblings

Most siblings of children who have ASDs fare well. Many even become quite helpful in the day-to-day functioning of the household. Some become great advocates for their siblings and even go on to choose professions that assist people with disabilities. But others may experience tremendous stress and resentment. Most siblings have a mix of emotions, feeling loving and supportive one minute, angry and bitter the next. Exactly how the typically developing children in a household respond to having a sibling with an ASD depends on the ages of the children and their maturity. It also depends on family dynamics.

Different children will have different concerns. Very young children are often worried about strange behaviors that scare or confuse them. Some children may be afraid of being the target of their sibling's anger and aggression. Others may try to compensate for the things that their siblings can't do. Some children are jealous over the attention that their sibling receives from their parents. Others may be frustrated at not being able to engage in a relationship with their sibling.

Teenagers may be concerned about what the future holds for their sibling with an ASD. They may worry about the role they'll need to play in caring for their sibling. Other children may wonder how to explain ASDs to their friends and feel embarrassed by their sibling's unusual behaviors and social deficits. Still others may become worried about their parents' stress and grief. Whatever emotions your typical child expresses, respect those feelings, however uncomfortable they may be to you.

Having open and honest discussions about autism at a level and in a way that your children can understand is critical to helping the siblings of a child with an ASD. If you do not tell your other children about their sibling's ASD, they may feel increasingly isolated or confused. But don't just offer one conversation or discussion about autism. Keep talking about it with your children as they grow up. When they are younger they might not understand the term ASD, but you can start by talking about the differences that other children may

---

A SISTER'S STORY: SHAY

"Being a sibling of someone with autism has been a great experience for me. My little brother, who was diagnosed with autism when he was 22 months old, is 9 years younger than me. I am the closest sibling to his age. I have taken on a caregiver role on my own accord since he was born. I always felt a special bond with him despite his lack of communication through words. From a young age he would come to me and guide me to what he wanted. I considered him a best friend, not a chore.

"Having a brother with autism has opened my eyes to the challenges and blessings of the families in the world of special needs people. He has been a source of joy for me as I have watched him make great strides in his communication skills. I cried with my mom when I came back from my first year in college and heard him count to 10 on his own at the age of 9. He has made me laugh with his excellent singing skills, belting out 'Reflection' from *Mulan* with such passion and exuberance. Although it has been hard to watch him struggle to communicate his complicated feelings, and I sometimes feel helpless trying to find him the help he needs, I would never trade the lessons I have learned from him. In his simple way, he has taught me what is important in life over the years by being my brother and friend."

have and about what it means to have a disability. You could even read books with them that have some characters with disabilities. Listen carefully to their concerns, which will certainly change over time.

It's also important to foster a relationship among siblings. Children who have ASDs typically have challenges with social skills. Siblings may give up when they can't engage them in interactions. But siblings can be taught simple ways to engage a child with an ASD and with time can provide a natural way for children with ASDs to work on their social skills.

Promote Sibling Harmony

Parents can ease the burden on siblings by trying to set aside some time to be alone with each of their children. It may be as little as a few minutes before bedtime or as much as a weekly afternoon outing. And remember the important events in all your children's lives. If your child with an ASD can't attend another child's graduation, find someone to be with him so you can still go.

Do the best you can to try and set reasonable expectations of your child with an ASD as you do with your other children in terms of chores and personal responsibilities. Doing so will not only help your child with an ASD develop the skills he needs to live as independently as possible; it will also help to dispel any notions of unfair treatment by siblings. Of course, being fair does not always mean equal responsibilities for all children. You will need to have ongoing talks with siblings about the challenges that autism brings for their sibling with an ASD and how they need to be understanding.

Finally, try to model a healthy perspective. How you view your child's ASD can be a source of strength for other family members. By seeking out information and support, you are showing your other children how to be strong and resilient in the face of a challenging circumstance. Also, by dwelling on the positive aspects of parenting your child with an ASD, you model the behavior that you want your other children to show toward those with disabilities.

A PARENT'S STORY: JENNIFER

For years, Jennifer was a single mother of 3 boys, all with autism. After a difficult divorce and having little support, she did the best she could to navigate the system of services for children with autism spectrum disorders alone. "I drove them to 17 therapies a week, cut the tags out of all their clothes, and confronted all their issues. I worried all the time. When would my oldest son talk and make friends? Why was my middle son biting himself? When would my youngest finally sleep through the night?

"Everything changed when I met and married my second husband. He has 4 children of his own. All are high achievers, athletically gifted, and socially successful. I wondered how the 7 were going to get along under one roof.

"Turns out, they get along great. Some of the issues are mine. For instance, having my stepchildren around accentuates for me all the challenges that my children still face. My step-kids get to do all kinds of stuff that my kids don't get to do, like going to birthday parties and having endless play-dates. They see what life is like every day for 'normal' kids. I can't really give that to them because we are still trying to learn stuff like how to talk and how to try a new food once in a while. It really breaks my heart.

"On the other hand, having 4 new older siblings who are super-functional has been outstanding for my kids. They have social peer models and language models now. They have extra help doing stuff that Mommy doesn't have extra time for, like learning to ride a bike and tie their shoes. It's awesome. In the few short months since we have moved in together, my kids have made the most gains ever in all areas of development. My stepchildren are the greatest gift in the world to me and to my sons."

Dealing With Your Own Stress

Raising a child with an ASD creates challenges on many levels. For many parents, there is stress in confronting their early concerns about behavior and development and then trying to find answers as to why their child is developing differently than other children. Some parents may have suspected autism all along but had no idea of the implications until they started doing research. Either way, most parents go through a lot of emotions as they come to terms with their child's diagnosis. In fact, a study at Eastern Michigan University found that families generally view a diagnosis of autism as a life-altering event that may initially lead to feelings of guilt and sadness, along with worry for their child's future. These emotions can lead many parents to feel overwhelmed.

After the diagnosis, the day-to-day challenges of autism can be stressful too. Successfully confronting the difficult moments that come with raising a child with a disability can tax even the most patient parents. Many of the challenges that affect children with ASDs can also affect caregivers. If your child struggles with sleep, for example, you will likely lose sleep in your effort to help your child.

Staying positive in the face of ASDs can be difficult, especially in the beginning when there is so much uncertainty about the future. In the face of this stress, you may find that you see less of your friends, spend less time with your spouse or other children, and do less of the things you enjoy. In some cases, you may even have to reduce your work hours or leave your job. The emotional and financial effect of these changes in your life can compound your stress. Some people have been known to develop mental health issues such as anxiety and depression.

While it may seem easy for outsiders to say and harder for you to do, try to find support from friends, other family members, and other families who are raising a child with an ASD. Studies have found that parents who seek support from other parents and community organizations generally have less stress. While all parents are different, many find support, understanding, and friendship when they join a parent support group in the community. Meetings with other families can be a major source of comfort and an excellent opportunity for networking. You can find some of these organizations in Chapter 9 and in Appendix A. Likewise, enrolling your child in a program appropriate for those with special needs (also known as adaptive recreation) allows you to meet other parents of children with disabilities and to share in the joys of watching your children participate.

Taking a break from your caregiving duties can go a long way toward reducing your stress. If family members aren't available, you may consider looking for respite services. Respite services provide care to your child while you take a break from those duties to attend to other family responsibilities or take some time off. While large cities may have respite services

---

IT'S OK TO ASK FOR HELP

For some people, the stress, anxiety, or depression can become overwhelming. If that happens to you, you may want to consider talking to a therapist. With a therapist, you should be able to talk honestly about everything you're feeling and experiencing—the good, the bad, and the ugly. Marriage or family therapy can also help work out challenges. To find a good therapist, talk to other parents or look for mental health organizations in your community for a referral.

A GOOD READ

The book *You Will Dream New Dreams* by Stanley D. Klein, PhD, and Kim Schive is a collection of essays written by parents of children with disabilities and conveys 4 key messages.

- You are not alone on this journey.

- The range of difficult feelings you have—and will continue to have—are a normal part of the human experience. We too have survived, and our lives have continued. You can go on and grow.

- Although there are no easy answers, you will find ways to cope. You are likely to discover inner resources you did not know existed.

- There is sadness; some dreams are lost. You will mourn, but you can heal. You will be happy again and you will dream new dreams.

---

readily available, it may be harder to find respite in small communities. Some respite services can be funded with help from Home and Community-Based Services Waiver programs (see Chapter 10). If there is any possibility you think you'll need respite in the future, apply for the waiver as soon as possible. Many of these waivers have waiting periods.

Taking Care of You

Mothers, in particular, are vulnerable to the stress of raising a child with an ASD. It often results from social isolation, financial burdens, and difficulties obtaining services. That's why it's so important to take care of yourself as well as your family. Here are some things you can do to guard against stress.

- *Build exercise into your life.* The time involved in raising a child with an ASD can be emotionally intense and all-consuming. One of the best ways to take care of yourself is to exercise. Regular physical activity gives you the physical and mental energy that can help you cope. Exercise is also critical to good health, maintaining a healthy weight, and keeping depression at bay. Of course, squeezing in a lengthy workout isn't always easy. Try to build movement into your day instead by taking short walks and exercising in front of the TV.

- *Devote time to being with friends.* One of the most important ways to reduce your stress is to spend time with friends. A weekly lunch or quick coffee break can nourish, energize, and revitalize you. It's also helpful to spend time with people in the autism community, especially other parents who can know exactly what you are experiencing.

- *Get educated about autism.* As the parent of a child with an ASD, it's critical to know not only the medical facts but also the laws, resources, and services surrounding autism. Having this information gives you a distinct advantage when it comes time to advocate for your child. It also gives you the knowledge and confidence you need to cope with challenging situations. As the saying goes, knowledge is power.

- *Become a planner.* Being a parent often means playing a variety of roles. One minute, you're a cook; the next you're a driver. When you have a child with an ASD, your responsibilities multiply considerably. Often you're also a therapist, an advocate, and a researcher. To better manage these roles, it helps to become skilled at planning. Knowing what's coming up in your schedule allows you to better maintain the routine and structure that most children with ASDs crave, which will lessen their anxiety—and yours.

- *Be on the lookout for depression.* Look for it in your spouse too. Depression isn't just feeling sad or unhappy. It's a serious mood disorder that alters your ability to function and makes it hard to enjoy everyday activities. Depression is common among people caring for children with ASDs. In fact, a study from the June 2010 issue of the *American Journal of Psychiatry* found that 26% of caregivers of children with autism develop depression. If you're having a hard time and think you're suffering from depression, talk to your doctor.

- *Get your sleep.* One of the best buffers against depression, stress, and fatigue is a good night's sleep. Do what you can to get your rest, even if it means taking a brief nap during the day. Try to go to bed and get up at the same time every day. Don't go overboard with caffeine late in the day. And try to relax before you crawl into bed.

A PARENT'S STORY: CHERYL

"We are finally going to see our older son who lives in San Diego with his wife and little boy. We decide to take our younger son who has autism. He might like to swim and go to SeaWorld. The only time he has flown was to go to Disneyland a couple of times, and it went OK.

"I make the mistake of telling him we are going on the airplane a week or so before we are leaving. He says, 'Airplane, airplane,' every 15 minutes for a couple of days, then starts adding, 'Disneyland, airplane,' the rest of the week. I say, 'No, we aren't going to Disneyland this time.' Perhaps he thinks if he says it enough times it will be true.

"We make the usual accommodations for the airplane ride: a backpack full of DVDs, the player charged up, the iPod with Disney music, books, candy, and Benadryl. I sit next to my son and my husband sits in front of him so that when he kicks the back of the seat the whole way there it doesn't annoy a stranger. We put the T-shirt on my son that says, 'I have autism, be nice to my mom,' so that we can hopefully avoid the stink eye and get a small amount of compassion.

"We make it to San Diego without a huge amount of distress, still hearing 'Disneyland' every so often. At SeaWorld, he is so afraid that we really might not be going to Disneyland that he can barely enjoy it. He does like the rides and the whales, but we have to buy him a new shirt when his gets wet because he cannot be wearing a wet shirt. The next day he throws in a couple 'SeaWorld's with the 'Disneyland' to break up the monotony.

"The ride home is priceless. Disneyland does not happen, so getting through the airport is distressing. He is ticked. We find the airport waiting area for our flight. He tries to get out the emergency exit door at the airport, setting off the alarm. The police come. The alarm goes off for a long, long time. Talk about sensory overload. We get in line to board, the long, long, very slowly moving line. It's like trying to contain a rabid cat inside 2 painted lines. People are getting as agitated as we are.

"'Why do they board first class first?' I wonder as the passengers are getting smacked by this flailing boy, their preflight martinis spilling everywhere. He starts to say, '14, 14, 14,' which was the row we were on leaving for San Diego. I say, 'No, we are in 13 this time. Look, 13, 13, 13.' We get into row 13, finally, and he climbs over row 13 to get into row 14.

"'Hmmm,' I say, 'maybe we should trade seats with these people?' He is biting me now and crying. The stewardess says, 'Oh, don't bite!' That was like telling a newborn not to cry or a dog not to shed. I pull out the DVD player, my pinch hitter, and to my dismay, the battery is dead. Now I'm questioning if there really is a God. So just to be sure, my husband and I both start praying, 'Please, please, make him go to sleep...' and then a miracle happens. He falls asleep.

"Next time we are going to Disneyland."

DO YOU HAVE DEPRESSION?

Depression is a common mood disorder that strikes 9% of all adults in the United States, the majority of them women. Depression is usually treated with medications, therapy, or a combination of both. According to the National Institute of Mental Health, the signs and symptoms are

- Persistent sad, anxious, or "empty" feelings

- Feelings of hopelessness or pessimism

- Feelings of guilt, worthlessness, or helplessness

- Irritability, restlessness

- Loss of interest in activities or hobbies once pleasurable, including sex

- Fatigue and decreased energy

- Difficulty concentrating, remembering details, and making decisions

- Insomnia, early-morning wakefulness, or excessive sleeping

- Overeating or appetite loss

- Thoughts of suicide, suicide attempts

- Persistent aches or pains, headaches, cramps, or digestive problems that do not ease even with treatment

---

- *Learn to accept help.* When a friend offers to help you out, tell her what you need. Maybe it's spending an hour with your child so you can take a walk, or driving your other child to a soccer game. Whatever it is, don't be afraid to tap your family or friends for some assistance. And make sure to enlist your spouse's help. Studies have found that most mothers derive a lot of emotional support and practical help from a spouse who is an equal partner.

- *Look for the joys in raising your child.* In spite of all the challenges, many parents say that raising a child with an ASD can be thrilling and exciting, especially when your child strives and reaches his potential. To truly appreciate any progress, however, often requires reframing your situation and changing your perspective. Altering your outlook can go a long way in helping you cope with the challenges of autism. Look for ways to define your experiences more positively. Doing so may give you greater confidence and strength.

Resilience

The standard assumption until the 1980s was that having a child with a disability would result in ongoing family suffering. This premise was challenged as researchers began to focus on family strengths, coping skills, and families' positive views of their child and themselves. Families, it was found, could be highly resilient. They are able to respond with strengths that transform them from merely surviving to actually thriving as they face the challenges of raising a child with special needs.

Research studies have identified the following characteristics in parents who successfully adapt to raising a child with a disability:

- Pleasure in providing care for their child
- Seeing their child as a source of joy
- Accomplishment in having done their best for their child
- Strengthened family relationships as result of collective response to the child's condition
- A new sense of purpose in life
- Increased spirituality
- New perspective on what is important in life

According to researchers from the Interactive Autism Network (IAN), "Parents told us they had come through the distress and grief of the initial diagnosis to adjust, celebrate their child and thrive." One parent told IAN, "He has taught us a lot about what's important in life." Another parent commented, "We decided not to let ASD be all our family was about."

Families who have successfully navigated the journey of raising a child with an ASD have redefined their circumstances, celebrate their child's specialness and gains, embrace a new outlook on life, and appreciate their daily pursuits in new ways.

Final Word

Learning your child has an ASD can certainly change your perception of what you thought your life might be. You may have to restructure your priorities and develop new coping skills. And you may have to change some of your plans for the future. But in their place will be new dreams, new goals, and new priorities. The key is finding ways to adapt and adjust that suit your family, your needs, and your circumstances. It likely won't be easy. But people often find strength from within and from those around them to succeed. By loving your child dearly, you will be inspired to do what you can to learn as much as possible about ASDs so that you too will be rewarded as you discover what works for your family.

Autism Champion: Jennifer Wood

Jennifer Wood of Plainfield, IL, can still remember the first time she went to bat for her son Tripp, who is now 10 years old. "The public special education preschool program would not furnish my 3-year-old with a car seat on the bus," she says. "I searched online until I found applicable statutes, codes, and case law, and I presented these to the school administration, along with a not-empty threat that I would hire a lawyer to ensure my son's safety."

The school listened. "Not only did he have a proper safety harness, but there was one ready and waiting on the first day of school 2 years later for my middle son, and another after that for my third son," she said. "My advocacy for my son in the first case solved the problem for all 3 of my sons."

For Jennifer, who spent years as a single mother raising 3 boys with ASDs, the incident marked the beginning of her work as a parent advocate. She began speaking at support group meetings for parents of children with special needs and became a volunteer mediator at Individualized Education Program meetings for other families. She also joined the Run for Autism program of the Organization for Autism Research (OAR) and began raising money by running marathons. She spent a year as the OAR national spokesperson while working as a volunteer mediator. She recently ended her volunteer work to pursue a law degree with a focus on ASD and the law.

For someone well-versed in the challenges of raising children with ASDs, Jennifer says getting a child in therapy is the key—along with a healthy dose of patience. "Therapy is a marathon, not a sprint," she says. She also recommends that parents talk to each other for support. "This journey is lonely enough," she says. "Do not travel it alone if you don't have to."

CHAPTER 14

The Future of Autism Spectrum Disorders

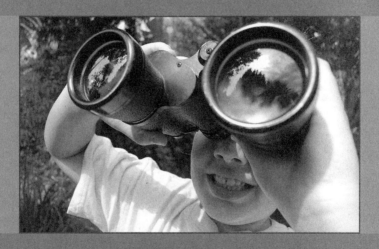

We've come a long way since the days when Bruno Bettelheim blamed cold, unloving mothers for their child's autism. Gone too are the days when autism was considered a form of schizophrenia, and many children with autism were separated from their parents and placed in institutions.

These days, we know a lot more about autism spectrum disorders (ASDs) than we ever have before. The rapid surge in the number of people who have been diagnosed with ASDs has made autism a critical area of research. At the same time, it has generated an important need to improve our understanding of this disorder, improve services for people with ASDs and their families, and given rise to federal and state laws and regulations designed to empower and protect people with autism, including the right to early intervention services, an appropriate education, and job training. People who have ASDs and their families have even become a political force. Clearly, autism has become a topic of intense focus and research in our society, which bodes well for creating opportunities for people who have the condition.

In spite of all these strides, there is still far to go in terms of understanding ASDs—why they occur, genetic and environmental risk factors, and what can be done to treat the individual and support the family. There are still many gaps in services, particularly for underrepresented segments of our population and for older adults with ASDs. The fact that these disorders vary so widely also warrants more attention if we are to provide children and adults with the best treatment. Keep in mind that autism spans a large spectrum and includes people who are nonverbal and rely on supports to help them meet the demands of their daily routines, as well as those who eventually secure full-time jobs and live independently.

In this chapter, we'll talk about the gains we've made in improving our understanding of ASDs, securing more protections for people with ASDs, and providing more services. We'll also examine what still needs to be done. Where do we go from here? What kinds of research are we looking at? How do we do a better job of serving the autism community?

Federal Leadership

In 2006, the US Congress passed the Combating Autism Act (CAA), which was intended to speed up ASD research and improve services for people with ASDs and their families. The legislation authorized the federal government to intensify the work it was doing on ASD research, surveillance, prevention, treatment, and education. It also resulted in appropriations of $924 million during the subsequent 5 fiscal years and increased federal spending on autism by at least 50%.

The CAA led to the creation of the Interagency Autism Coordinating Committee (IACC), which is made up of representatives from several agencies within the US Department of Health and Human Services, members of the public affected by autism, and participants in the autism advocacy and research community. The IACC reports to Congress on progress being made on ASD. Every year, the IACC publishes a strategic plan that outlines the conduct of autism research, creates a summary of advances in ASD research, and monitors federal activities related to ASDs.

The CAA helped to fund more surveillance and awareness programs under the US Centers for Disease Control and Prevention (CDC). Surveillance helps experts understand the *prevalence* of ASDs, or how many cases there are at any given time within the United States. Among these increased surveillance efforts was the reauthorization of the Autism and Developmental Disabilities Monitoring Network, which keeps tabs on the prevalence of

---

SIGNING THE COMBATING AUTISM ACT

"For the millions of Americans whose lives are affected by autism, today is a day of hope. The Combating Autism Act of 2006 will increase public awareness about this disorder and provide enhanced federal support for autism research and treatment. By creating a national education program for doctors and the public about autism, this legislation will help more people recognize the symptoms of autism. This will lead to early identification and intervention, which is critical for children with autism. I am proud to sign this bill into law and confident that it will serve as an important foundation for our nation's efforts to find a cure for autism."

President George W. Bush, December 19, 2006

ASDs throughout the United States. Gathering information about ASD prevalence helps identify trends in ASDs over time and may eventually help us understand who is at risk for ASDs. Let's look at some of the other key areas of interest.

Earlier and Better Diagnosis

One of the most important changes in recent history has been the emphasis on early diagnosis. Experts now know that the symptoms of ASDs can be reliably detected by the time a child is 3 years old, but that early signs can be seen as early as 12 months of age. Yet, according to a 2012 study, the average age of diagnosis is when a child is around 4 years old. Detecting autism early can make an enormous difference in how well a child fares in terms of treatment and therapies. To emphasize the importance of early diagnosis, the CDC has been promoting its "Learn the Signs. Act Early." campaign since 2004 to bolster autism awareness and encourage early diagnosis. The American Academy of Pediatrics now recommends screening all children for ASDs at 18 and 24 months of age.

While these efforts have made an enormous difference, much still needs to be done. Diagnosis continues to be difficult because so-called typical development varies widely in young children. For instance, some children speak at an early age, while others do not speak until much later and yet are still within the range of what's considered typical and appropriate. Diagnosis is also difficult because of widely varying screening and diagnostic practices across the United States.

Another challenge is the lack of access to services for children in certain socioeconomic groups. Children who come from disadvantaged backgrounds or live in rural communities may have more difficulty accessing quality health care or services. As a result, many of these children go undiagnosed or are diagnosed at a later age. Even those who are diagnosed may face prolonged waits until therapists are available to provide treatment. Efforts to build public awareness and improve early diagnosis and access to treatment services in these communities will require a better understanding of these socioeconomic disparities.

In addition, there are disparities in diagnosis among ethnic groups. African American and Hispanic children are generally diagnosed at a later age than white children. To address these differences, experts want to develop better, more reliable screening and diagnostic tools that are easy to administer to large populations and yet are effective in different groups, including girls, older children, and children who come from different ethnic and racial backgrounds.

Researchers are also hoping to find a reliable biomarker—a distinct biochemical, genetic, or molecular characteristic or substance—that identifies young children at risk for ASDs or who have an ASD. Ideally, the biomarker will be obvious before birth or shortly after. A reliable biomarker will allow for more accurate diagnosis. Without a biomarker, health care experts will continue to rely on observing behaviors that are often not apparent until well after birth, which creates a significant time lag. The delay in diagnosis is a missed opportunity for early intervention.

Addressing the Entire Spectrum

Almost everyone on the autism spectrum struggles with social skills, communication deficits, and stereotypic behaviors. But the diversity of behavioral problems and developmental challenges is broad. Some people with an ASD have a disability that significantly challenges their ability to communicate wants and needs, and so they rely more heavily on caregivers to help with activities of daily living. For others, their disability poses fewer challenges and they achieve a higher level of functioning.

The broadness of the autism spectrum—often referred to as its heterogeneity—not only represents the wide range of abilities and needs of those with the diagnosis but also the multiple underlying causes of ASDs, as discussed in Chapter 2. Such variability in function, associated medical conditions, and types of underlying brain differences has made it difficult for researchers to identify specific treatments that will lead to the best possible outcome in all individuals with an ASD. The diversity in symptoms and causes suggests that different people will respond differently to available interventions, be they behavioral, developmental, medical, or other. The key is knowing what intervention or combination of interventions will work best for whom and how to establish reasonable expectations for future functioning.

Addressing the needs of the entire spectrum also means looking at the needs of adolescents and adults with ASDs. Most people view ASDs as a childhood problem. In reality, the majority of children with ASDs do not outgrow their diagnosis. Their symptoms and needs simply change over time as they become adults. Currently, the needs of most adults are not being well addressed.

In the IACC *2011 Strategic Plan for Autism Spectrum Disorder Research,* the needs of adults were identified as an area that required more research, in particular practical strategies for improving quality of life and functioning among adolescents and adults. The goal is to help adolescents transition into adulthood and lead meaningful but self-determined lives with access to services they may still require.

Yet another gap is the low enrollment of girls in ASD research. Boys outnumber girls in research studies by a ratio of 4 to 1, in large part because the disorder is more common in boys than girls. But girls' participation is critical to understanding why ASDs are more common in boys. It may explain whether being a girl offers protection against ASDs, how gender may affect diagnosis, and how the disorder develops over time in girls as opposed to boys.

Research also needs to involve more low-functioning individuals. Right now, many studies favor the enrollment of high-functioning people, who tend to be more capable of participating and cooperating in studies. But findings from these studies may not apply to people with ASDs who face more significant language and cognitive challenges. More studies of people who have lower levels of function are required if we are to truly understand the cause of ASDs in all people on the spectrum. Additional studies will also help us to understand which treatments may be most beneficial to this group of individuals.

THE PUSH FOR INSURANCE COVERAGE

As any parent can tell you, the cost of autism can be difficult. To help families financially, advocacy groups—including the American Academy of Pediatrics and its state chapters—have been pushing hard for insurance coverage. To date, slightly more than half of all states have enacted legislation that requires some form of insurance coverage for children with autism. Details of the laws vary by state. Families, pediatricians, and other advocates continue to work with state lawmakers to improve existing laws and enact new policies to improve insurance coverage for children with autism.

Can Autism Spectrum Disorders Be Prevented?

Someday, in an ideal world, we'll be able to prevent ASDs. But before we can do that, it's critical that we understand the cause of ASDs. Most experts are fairly certain that ASDs, like many complex conditions, are the result of a genetic risk interacting with an environmental exposure. Identifying the specific genes and exposures involved, however, has not been easy. Most of the focus has been on genetics, including rare genetic mutations, chromosomal abnormalities, and deletions and duplications of genetic material. But each of these events accounts for a small percentage of cases, which suggests that multiple genes may be involved or that autism is the result of several genetic variations and combinations.

Most recently, researchers have been exploring epigenetics, the study of DNA changes in genetic expression as a result of exposure to something in the environment. Genes may be silenced or activated in response to environmental influences such as diet, stress, and exposure to toxins. No doubt, we can expect more research into epigenetics as a possible cause of ASDs.

Until recently, less emphasis had been placed on identifying specific environmental factors that may increase the risk for ASDs. The only environmental factor that has been heavily studied is vaccines. Many studies have now shown that vaccines do not cause autism (see Chapter 2). Other factors under study include parental age and exposure to infections, toxins, and other biological agents such as pesticides and pollutants. Future studies will look at environmental risk factors in the prenatal and early postnatal periods to help identify risks. Eliminating these risks, once they're identified, will hopefully go a long way toward preventing autism and reducing the numbers of people who have ASDs in future generations.

FAST FACT

In recent years, the amount of funding dedicated to autism research has surged. Back in 2000, the National Institutes of Health allocated about $50 million toward autism research. By 2010, that figure had jumped to $217 million. Interest in autism research is also reflected in the rising number of medical journals dedicated specifically to autism, including *Autism, Autism Research and Treatment,* and the *Journal of Autism and Developmental Disorders.*

Improving Treatment

Finding the best treatment for someone with an ASD remains a significant challenge, largely because the biology of autism continues to be so incompletely understood. Though ASDs are classified as developmental brain disorders, the exact neurologic abnormality remains unknown. It's also unclear why some children regress. As young toddlers they meet major developmental milestones such as language, social, and communication skills, only to lose them and be diagnosed with ASDs or another disorder. We currently know that there are numerous causes of ASDs. That may mean that certain people will respond better to specific treatments. Efforts are underway, for example, in conditions such as fragile X syndrome and neurofibromatosis type 1, to test specific medications looking for a disease-specific response to treatment. This type of approach may expand considerably in the future.

Knowing which treatments work best in which people will require a lot more research. With the exception of applied behavior analysis (see Chapter 4), most treatments now in use are not backed by solid scientific evidence from randomized, controlled trials, which are considered the gold standard of scientific research. But as noted in Chapter 7, just because a treatment doesn't have scientific evidence backing it up does not mean it doesn't work; it simply means that scientists haven't subjected the treatment to rigorous scientific study.

The research on treatments is twofold. For one thing, we need to find new treatments that target events occurring at the molecular level in children with ASDs. Developing these targeted treatments will most likely require finding biomarkers in plasma, saliva, or cerebrospinal fluid, or tissue that will help reveal children who are at risk for ASDs. Discovering a reliable biomarker, in turn, will offer hope for prevention. The other aspect of treatment research needs to test is how well existing treatments actually work. Many of these are already in use, but evidence of their usefulness is often anecdotal and descriptive, not scientific and quantitative.

Scientists need to do more research into coexisting conditions that are common in ASDs, such as epilepsy, gastrointestinal disorders, and sleep issues. There needs to be a better understanding of how treatments for these conditions may affect the core symptoms of autism as well as how these treatments may affect the overall function of the individual.

THE ULTIMATE INTERVENTION?

At the moment, there is no cure for autism spectrum disorders (ASDs), though children with ASDs can certainly progress developmentally and learn new skills. Our scientific understanding of the cause of ASDs is far from complete. The American Academy of Pediatrics strongly supports ongoing studies funded through the Centers for Disease Control and Prevention and the National Institutes of Health that are trying to determine the underlying biology of and factors in our modern environment that may be responsible for autism.

At the same time, more studies are needed on pharmacologic treatments and dietary supplements for those with ASDs. So far, the US Food and Drug Administration has only approved risperidone and aripiprazole for treating irritability and aggression in some children with ASDs. And many people with ASDs are already using dietary supplements, despite the lack of hard science behind them. Developing new treatments that are more targeted will provide not only more options for treatment but also a better understanding of the safety and effectiveness of these treatments.

Support for Research

Extensive research on ASDs still needs to be done, and it will require significant collaboration, money, and manpower. For it to be successful, the field will require researchers to share more data, which will improve their analyses of the information gathered. Collecting this information will help researchers determine whether early diagnosis and services, as well as the types of services, affect the course of an individual's ASD.

To enhance research efforts, scientists also need more human tissue. These tissues and samples will need to come not only from people with ASDs but also from people who do not have the disorder for comparison. Developing methods and procedures for storing and accessing these specimens will be critical to the process too.

In addition, research will require more surveillance. Closely observing autism over time will help experts track the numbers of children with ASDs and any trends in how often it occurs. It will also help identify potential risk factors. Information gleaned from this surveillance may be used to improve early diagnosis, education and health services, and community programs.

Future research must examine the delivery of services, including the economics. For instance, we need to determine the cost benefits of providing the most effective treatments. We must answer critical questions such as, what are the costs and potential long-term savings when we help a child become more independent and functional in today's world? Should we be investing more up front to realize greater benefits down the road? What are the most economic models for providing the greatest benefit to the greatest number of children?

We also need more information on how to best deliver the services to the people who need them. How do we provide the most appropriate and effective therapies to the greatest number of people? Are we doing that right now? And if not, what are the barriers that are preventing us?

At the same time, we need to look to the future and assess whether we have the manpower to handle the growing numbers of children being diagnosed with ASDs. Researchers should do a needs analysis and compare with the numbers of professionals working in the field. We must analyze whether training programs of today are producing enough new professionals for the future. And if not, what can we do to encourage today's youth to pursue careers in these areas of need? How can we entice colleges and universities to increase their student capacity to accommodate the increased demand?

Other important areas of focus include communicating new knowledge about ASDs and training researchers. Translating information gleaned from research and communicating it to professionals and the public will allow new and worthwhile findings to be turned into practice for people with ASDs and their families. The field will also need more scientists trained in doing autism research, in particular interdisciplinary research.

There are ways that you can help in the efforts to learn more about ASDs. If you have a child with an ASD or have autism yourself, you may want to consider participating in research studies. (Go to www.nimh.nih.gov to participate or learn about federally and privately funded clinical trials.) The information you provide may be critical to building our understanding of this complex disorder. This may lead to much-needed improvements in the evaluation and treatment of ASDs as well as services for people who have it and their families.

CHAPTER 15

Advocating for Children With Autism Spectrum Disorders

All parents are advocates whenever they speak out on behalf of their children. But for parents of children who have autism spectrum disorders (ASDs), advocacy can often go beyond your child to become a personal crusade in a world still struggling to understand these neurologic disorders and how to accommodate people who have needs associated with them.

The dictionary defines *advocate* as someone who strongly and publicly supports someone or something. You'd be hard pressed to find people with stronger opinions about autism than parents of children who have ASDs. These days, parents are at the forefront of autism advocacy. Many become impassioned about autism after they struggle to meet the needs of their own children. Others find themselves doing endless amounts of research into autism and then becoming committed to sharing that knowledge and putting it to good use. Still others want to promote a particular message about an aspect of autism. The good news is, autism organizations are more than eager to tap into the energy and drive that these advocate parents bring to the cause.

Throughout this book, you've read profiles of people who are advocates for autism. But you can make a difference too by getting involved in your local school, hometown community, or nonprofit groups. In this chapter, we'll take a look at what it takes to be an advocate and the many ways you can get involved. Maybe you will find inspiration in these pages to become an advocate yourself.

What Advocates Do

Advocates, first and foremost, are educators. They're in the public teaching people about ASDs, what they are and how they affect lives. Advocates may be teaching lawmakers about the importance of autism-related legislation, helping parents understand their rights under special education law, or educating the community about ASDs. Advocates aren't shy about taking a position and persuading others to understand the value of their stance, whether they're trying to convince the school board that a new special education teacher is needed or asking politicians for more money to fund autism research.

WHY ADVOCACY?

Advocacy at the community, state, or federal level can make a meaningful and lasting difference to children in your community and state and nationwide. Community, state, and federal advocacy allows you to become part of a broader network of advocates that works systemically to raise awareness, educate, and create policies that can help keep children safe and healthy.

For many people, becoming an advocate starts with identifying an unmet need and having the desire to make changes to improve the situation. For others, advocacy grows out of genuine concern and kindness for those less fortunate. Others may see advocacy as a way to show appreciation for the opportunities they have received, a chance for them to pay it forward.

And advocacy, on any level, doesn't need to be done on a grand scale or performed over the course of an entire lifetime. Plenty of people have found smaller causes in their own communities and have turned them into worthwhile pursuits. The key to finding your cause is to tap into your passion, to find what matters most to you. For many people, that passion rests with their children and other loved ones.

FAST FACT

Parents aren't the only ones advocating on behalf of children with autism spectrum disorders. Pediatricians and other physicians, teachers, administrators, therapists, and special education providers also get involved in doing advocacy work.

One of the most important things to do before you get out there is to have a clear goal in mind. What exactly do you want? What is your role as the advocate? How will you get there? Sometimes it takes time to figure out what your immediate goal is. But if you have a long-term plan, it may help shape what you do now.

Required Skills

Anyone can sound off with her views in a meeting, on a blog, or in a letter. But effective advocates possess skills that allow them to make their points clearly and precisely, with the goal of persuading others—and getting the results they seek. Here are some of the skills that these effective advocates display.

EUNICE KENNEDY SHRIVER

Among the most well-known advocates for the disabled was Eunice Kennedy Shriver, who launched Special Olympics. Mrs Shriver was the sister of President John F. Kennedy and Senator Edward M. Kennedy of Massachusetts. Her passion for the disabled grew out of her love for her sister Rosemary, the eldest daughter of Joseph Kennedy and his wife Rose.

As a child, Rosemary was slow to crawl, walk, and speak. Once in school it was apparent she had an intellectual disability, and as a young woman she grew increasingly agitated and suffered from violent mood swings. Unable to care for herself, Rosemary spent the rest of her life in an institution, where she received the daily care she needed, until her death at the age of 86.

Mrs Shriver had deep compassion for her older sister and the challenges that Rosemary faced throughout her life. In 1962, she started a day camp for young people with intellectual disabilities in her backyard that she called Camp Shriver. She wanted to see the children use their skills in a variety of sports and physical activities. The camp grew in popularity. Six years later, the first International Special Olympics Summer Games were held in Chicago, IL. Eunice Kennedy Shriver promised that this new organization would give children with intellectual disabilities the chance to play, compete, and grow. Today, the Special Olympics are held in 170 countries and serve more than 4 million people.

But Mrs Shriver did not stop there. She also took over leadership of the Joseph P. Kennedy, Jr. Foundation, an organization founded to honor her oldest brother Joseph, who was killed in World War II. According to the Special Olympics Web site (www.specialolympics.org), the foundation has 2 goals: to seek the prevention of intellectual disability by identifying its causes, and to improve the means by which society deals with citizens who have intellectual disabilities.

Mrs Shriver worked tirelessly on behalf of people with intellectual disabilities. She helped to launch the National Institute of Child Health and Human Development in 1962. She also helped establish the Eunice Kennedy Shriver Intellectual and Developmental Disabilities Research Centers and the University Affiliated Facilities, now known as University Centers for Excellence in Developmental Disabilities. Her efforts to develop clinical training programs for professionals working with children with disabilities and special health care needs have evolved into the Leadership Education in Neurodevelopmental and Related Disabilities programs.

Eunice Kennedy Shriver died in 2009, leaving behind a legacy of work on behalf of the disabled.

- *They know how to do research and gather facts.* Advocates gather facts and information. As they gather information and organize documents and records, they learn about a child's disability and educational history. Advocates use facts and independent documentation to work with schools and education officials to achieve appropriate services and outcomes for their children.
- *They become familiar with the players in their school, community, or organization.* Advocates know how decisions are made, and they know who makes them.
- *They know about their legal rights.* Advocates stay on top of special education laws, regulations, and cases involving children with special needs. They also know the procedures to follow to protect their rights and children's rights.
- *They always arrive prepared.* Advocates are planners who go to meetings, presentations, and other events with all the key information they need. They prepare ahead of time and know their objectives before they go. They also know whom they need to approach and influence.
- *They ask questions and are good listeners.* Advocates know they sometimes have to probe for answers and aren't afraid to ask questions, even if the answer seems obvious.
- *They are record keepers.* Information is critical in the world of advocacy work, so smart advocates always keep documents on hand. They also take extensive notes and write follow-up letters if they have lingering questions or to confirm what happened at a meeting.
- *They put their energy into finding solutions, not assigning blame.* Looking for someone to blame accomplishes nothing. Advocates prefer instead to spend their precious time seeking solutions to their problems. They do it using the knowledge they acquire.
- *They aren't afraid to tell their stories.* Putting a face on a policy issue or while seeking a solution to a challenge taps into the hope and potential of an advocate's personal experience and can help bring about meaningful change.
- *They know how to get their point across without being confrontational.* They are good communicators who have learned the art of negotiation and mastered understanding when it's important to talk and to listen. They realize the importance of making everyone feel like they "win" in some way, if possible.

> "For all those whose cares have been our concern, the work goes on, the cause endures, the hope still lives, and the dream shall never die."
>
> **Senator Edward Moore "Ted" Kennedy, August 12, 1980**

Types of Advocacy Work

The word *advocate* is broad for a simple reason: there's a lot you can do. It can be as basic as writing a check to support autism research or as involved as creating an autism support group in your community. It can be lobbying state legislators for reforms to help people with ASDs, writing articles about autism in your local newspaper, or volunteering for an organization to stuff envelopes. The possibilities for involvement are endless but always start from the same place: love for your child and concern for her well-being.

As we've already noted, most people who become advocates discover their passion while working on behalf of their own children. If they're successful, they may feel empowered and want to get involved so they can help improve the lives of other children. The next thing they know, they are involved in the local chapter of an autism organization, participating in a walk to raise money, or writing letters to their congressional representatives on behalf of people who have ASDs. Others become involved when a friend encourages them to take up the cause.

If you think you'd like to do advocacy work in the field of autism, consider your passion, talents, and interests. Consult the resources in Appendix A and talk to others in your community. You'll be amazed at all the ways you can help out.

Can I Do It?

Anyone can be an advocate. The most important thing to do as an advocate is to become well-versed in the topic. Knowledge is power. So read about ASDs and special education laws and stay informed about related legislation. Find out how other organizations raise money or create awareness. Talk to others who know what you need to learn. Subscribe to appropriate magazines and journals. Keep up to date on ongoing developments, and network and share information with other individuals and groups.

At this point you might be saying you're too shy, too easily intimidated, or too scared to be an advocate. No doubt, being an advocate takes a degree of confidence and courage. For some people, that can come naturally. With others, it might take more effort and time. No matter where you stand right now, your confidence in advocating will grow over time. Each time you get results, no matter how small or big, you'll feel that much more empowered to speak out. Just remember, no one knows your story better than you.

If you do decide to pursue advocacy work, don't overlook your own needs in the process. Raising children with ASDs takes an excessive amount of time, energy, and patience. Add jobs, home maintenance, and advocacy into the mix and you'll probably feel a bit overwhelmed. If you become an advocate, make sure to take time for yourself to recharge and renew. For many parents, advocating allows them to feel like they are able to take some control of a situation and diagnosis in which there is very little.

The Road Ahead

By reading this book, you have gained a solid base of information on how to raise a child with an ASD. But acquiring knowledge shouldn't stop here. Autism has become a major public health concern and as a result, the field is constantly evolving. Staying on top of the latest research and developments will help you be the best possible parent and advocate.

Parenting a child with an ASD isn't easy. There will be days when you want to cry, scream, and throw your own tantrum. There will be many moments when you are tired and worn out. But there will also be many days when you celebrate and rejoice in all that your child has accomplished and how far you and your family have come. We hope this book, while helping you to understand and face the challenges, above all helps provide more opportunity for you to acknowledge and embrace the joyous moments and unique gifts that appear in your journey.

Autism Champion: Cheryl C. Smith

As the mother of a young child with severe autism, Cheryl C. Smith was unsure how she could afford to send her son Carson to a special school. "His kindergarten tuition at the Carmen B. Pingree Center for Children with Autism was more than my son's tuition in medical school at the University of Utah," she recalls.

Cheryl met with her state representative, J. Morgan Philpot, and he agreed to sponsor a bill. "I spent the next months doing interviews, sending letters and e-mails, making calls, talking to parents, taking tours, going up to the capitol," Cheryl recalls. "I worked on it for more than 50 hours a week while the session was in."

Her efforts paid off. In 2005, Utah became the first state in the United States to offer private school scholarships to children with special needs. It was named the Carson Smith Scholarship. "People approach me all the time teary eyed and tell me thanks for the work I did, they could not have their child in the place they need to be without the scholarship," Cheryl says. "Some were able to stay home with their other children, some to pay off that second mortgage they took out for their disabled child, some to reinstate their phone. But I didn't do it alone."

Cheryl became the president of the Autism Council of Utah. Carson started talking around age 9, his first heartwarming word, "Mom." Cheryl's advice on raising a child with an ASD: "Give yourself a break. We can't fix everything. Most things don't change no matter how long we cry or how much cookie dough we eat. The things that we deal with may or may not change, but we can always dig down to find the joy in ourselves."

Afterword

Shana's Special Wish

Written by Nicole Ashley Herzog

Age 9

This story is dedicated to all the Shana and Freddys of the world and to my brother Eli who doesn't understand how much I love and accept him just the way he is.

ໂ. ໂ. ໂ. ໂ. ໂ.

On a sweet little street lived a sweet little family; Mommy, Daddy, and Shana (that's me). We were as happy as can be, but I knew we would be even happier if I had a little brother or sister. Pretty much that's all I ever talked about. And whenever I made a wish, I always wished for the same thing. Like when we were at the mall, and I threw in the five pennies and one quarter that were at the bottom of my purse into the fountain, or the time when I blew out the candles on my birthday cake. I wished and wished. And do you know what happened? A miracle! After all my wishing, finally, a baby was on the way!

When the baby arrived, he was so cute—at least that's what everyone said. I thought he looked weird. He had plenty of wrinkles, just like my grandpa. But just the same, I loved my new little brother to pieces. He smiled at me and he was chubby, and he followed me with his eyes and became very excited whenever I came into the room. It was great. I loved to make him laugh by tickling him and playing Peek-a-boo.

Our life went on as usual. We were a sweet little family; Mommy, Daddy, Shana and Freddy. We were as happy as can be, except lately Mommy and Daddy had worried looks on their faces, and sometimes I saw Mommy crying.

"What's wrong, Mommy?" I asked. "Oh, Mommy's just a little sad, Shana. Nothing for you to worry about. Hey, how about some hot chocolate?" Mommy knows I love hot chocolate. Hot chocolate and coconut jelly beans always make me happy. "Yay! I'll get the mugs!"

One night as Freddy wobbly walked around in his "Here Comes Trouble" t-shirt and puffy diaper, he carried a little set of wooden numbers from my puzzle box. "Aw, isn't that cute, Mommy? Freddy likes my number puzzle." He walked around saying, "Eight! Seven!" And he held up the number six and turned it upside down and said, "Nine!" It was so wonderfully funny because Freddy hadn't really said any words up until that moment.

The thing is, Freddy started carrying those numbers around with him everywhere he went. And once when I pointed to a guitar and asked him "Hey, Freddy, what do you see?" He said, "Eight!" And do you know what? That guitar really did look like an eight. Suddenly, I realized Freddy didn't just like numbers. Freddy LOVED numbers. He especially loved the number eight. He even took Daddy's glasses off one day at the park and held them sideways. And guess what he said? That's right…Eight!

I caught myself starting to get annoyed with the kid. Eight this, eight that. "Yeah, ok, Freddy. We get it!" Because you see, I wanted to read to Freddy and be silly with Freddy and play school with Freddy. But all he cared about were those stinkin' numbers. Seventeen also seemed to make quite an impression on him. Hmm. One plus seven equals…eight. Ahhh!

Still, Freddy is as cute as a button. He has a little chubby face with big pink cheeks and a huge smile. But something is different about him. Mommy told me he has something called autism. "Autism? What's that Mommy? Is Freddy sick?" I asked. "No, Shana. He's not sick. But his little brain works very differently than other people's brains." I asked, "And is that why he loves numbers so much?" Mommy nodded yes, and her eyes became watery as she turned and smiled at Freddy who had just walked into the room with two straws, proudly showing us how he had bent one of them to make a seven.

At that moment, we both laughed. I hugged and kissed Freddy and made him play Ring-around-the Rosie. And do you know what? Freddy laughed and giggled, and he loved Ring-around-the Rosie

Like most kids, Freddy loves to play in the water and go down the water slide at the pool. But I notice Freddy never has any little friends who want to play with him. Sometimes that makes me sad because I wish Freddy did have friends, friends that will look past the funny noises he makes or the way he flaps his little hands when he's really excited. But that's ok, because Freddy has me, and I will always be his friend.

Recently Freddy has discovered other interests. He loves classical music, especially Mozart and Bach. Oh, and how could I forget his fascination with Christmas music. I remember one summer when it was a scorching 100 degrees outside and we had the air conditioner on full blast as "Jingle Bells" blared from Mommy's car radio. Luckily, that's the summer I got my iPod.

Even though Freddy isn't perfect, and he may not be the little brother I had wished for, I wouldn't trade him for all the coconut jelly beans in the world. Because I love Freddy, and he loves me…almost as much as he loves the number eight.

🐾 🐾 🐾 **END** 🐾 🐾 🐾

Appendixes

Resources

This is not an all-inclusive list; however, the following suggestions will help you get started in your search for information. Make sure your pediatrician knows about your questions and concerns; share the information you find in your research. Remember, you and your pediatrician are partners in your child's health.

Please note: Listing here does not imply an endorsement by the American Academy of Pediatrics (AAP). The AAP is not responsible for the content of the resources. Phone numbers and Web sites are as current as possible but may change at any time.

American Academy of Pediatrics Resources

American Academy of Pediatrics

847/434-4000

www.aap.org

Professional medical organization of more than 60,000 pediatricians dedicated to the physical, mental, and social health and well-being of infants, children, adolescents, and young adults

www.HealthyChildren.org

The official parenting Web site of the AAP

www.aap.org/autism

The AAP Council on Children With Disabilities (COCWD) is dedicated to optimal care and development of children with disabilities and to the support of their families within a medical home. The COCWD Autism Subcommittee serves as the main point of contact for the AAP on issues related to autism spectrum disorders (ASDs).

Government Web Sites

Centers for Disease Control and Prevention

800/CDC-INFO (232-4636)

www.cdc.gov/ncbddd/autism

Offers information about the prevalence of autism and trends in autism as well as the "Learn the Signs. Act Early." campaign

Maternal & Child Health Library at Georgetown University

877/624-1935

www.mchlibrary.info/KnowledgePaths/kp_autism.html

A selection of current, high-quality resources about ASD identification and intervention; separate sections identify resources about ASDs and environmental health research and concerns about vaccines.

National Center for Complementary and Alternative Medicine

888/644-6226

www.nccam.nih.gov

Lead agency for scientific research on complementary and alternative medicine

National Dissemination Center for Children with Disabilities

800/695-0285

www.nichcy.org

Information about laws, services, and research affecting children with disabilities, including autism

National Early Childhood Technical Assistance Center

www.nectac.org

Supported by the US Department of Education Office of Special Education Programs under the provisions of the Individuals with Disabilities Education Act

National Institute of Mental Health

866/615-6464

www.nimh.nih.gov

Information about ASDs, including news, clinical trials, and access to other Web sites

National Institute of Neurological Disorders and Stroke

800/352-9424

www.ninds.nih.gov/disorders/autism/autism.htm

Provides information about autism as well as organizations about autism

US Department of Education

202/884-8215

http://idea.ed.gov

Provides information about the federal laws ensuring services for children with disabilities

Educational and Therapeutic Organizations

Association for Behavioral Analysis International

269/492-9310

www.abainternational.org

Membership organization that develops, supports, and enhances the field of applied behavioral analysis

DIR/Floortime

301/656-2667

www.icdl.com

Among its objectives, the Developmental, Individual Difference, Relationship-based (DIR)/Floortime model includes building healthy foundations for social, emotional, and intellectual capacities rather than focusing on skills and isolated behaviors.

Responsive Teaching

216/368-1707

www.responsiveteaching.org

A parent-mediated program of instruction for children younger than 6 years that focuses on cognition, communication, and social-emotional functioning

The SCERTS Model

www.scerts.com

Focuses on children with challenges in social communication and emotional regulation

TEACCH Autism Program at the University of North Carolina School of Medicine

919/966-2174

www.teacch.com

Evidence-based program that uses structured teaching to work with people who have ASDs in building life skills

Other Associations and Resources

American Academy of Child & Adolescent Psychiatry

202/966-7300

www.aacap.org

Professional medical organization focused on the health and treatment of children affected by mental, behavioral, and developmental disorders

American Academy of Pediatrics National Center for Medical Home Implementation

www.medicalhomeinfo.org

The National Center for Medical Home Implementation is a cooperative agreement between the Maternal and Child Health Bureau and the AAP that provides medical home resources and advocacy materials, technical assistance, and tools to physicians, families, and other medical and nonmedical providers who care for children, including children with special needs.

Association for Science in Autism Treatment

www.asatonline.org

Organization that promotes the use of effective, science-based treatments for people with autism, regardless of age, severity of condition, income, or place of residence

Association of University Centers on Disabilities

301/588-8252

www.aucd.org

A resource for local, state, national, and international agencies, organizations, and policy makers concerned about people living with developmental and other disabilities and their families

Autism Science Foundation

212/391-3913

www.autismsciencefoundation.org

Helps support autism research and provides information about autism to the general public

Autism Society of America

800/3AUTISM (328-8476)

www.autism-society.org

Organization that strives to improve the lives of people affected by autism by providing information about services and the latest in treatment, education, research, and advocacy

Autism Speaks

212/252-8584

www.autismspeaks.org

Supports research into the causes, prevention, treatments, and a cure for autism; raising awareness of autism; and advocating for the needs of individuals with autism and their families

Consortium of Academic Health Centers for Integrative Medicine

612/624-9166

www.imconsortium.org

Aims to advance the principles and practices of integrative health care within academic institutions; includes 51 academic medical centers and affiliate institutions and provides membership with a community of support for its academic missions and a collective voice for influencing change

Easter Seals

800/221-6827

www.easterseals.com

Provides services for individuals with autism, developmental disabilities, physical disabilities, and other special needs as well as their families

Family Voices

888/835-5669

www.familyvoices.org

Aims to achieve family-centered care for all children and youth with special health care needs and/or disabilities

Interactive Autism Network

443/923-7330

www.iancommunity.org

Online project that brings together people affected by ASDs and researchers; goal is to facilitate research that will lead to advancements in understanding and treating ASDs

National Center for Family/Professional Partnerships

888/835-5669

www.fv-ncfpp.org

A project of Family Voices, promotes families as partners in the decision-making of health care for children and youth with special health care needs at all levels of care

National Health Care Transition Center

603/228-8111

www.gottransition.org

National resource that supports optimal transitions from pediatric to adult models of health care for youth with and without special health care needs

Organization for Autism Research

703/243-9710

www.researchautism.org

Focuses on applied research and how it provides tangible and practical benefits to people with autism and their families

Special Needs Alliance

www.specialneedsalliance.com

National not-for-profit organization of attorneys dedicated to the practice of disability and public benefits law; connects individuals with disabilities, their families, and their advisors with nearby attorneys who focus their practices in the disability law arena

Special Olympics

800/700-8585

www.specialolympics.org

Provides children and adults with intellectual disabilities year-round sports training and athletic competition in a variety of Olympic-type sports to develop physical fitness, demonstrate courage, experience joy, and participate in a sharing of gifts, skills, and friendship with their families, other Special Olympics athletes, and the community

Books

General

Attwood T. *The Complete Guide to Asperger's Syndrome.* London, England: Jessica Kingsley Publishers; 2007

Bashe PR, Kirby BL. *The OASIS Guide to Asperger Syndrome: Advice, Support, Insight, and Inspiration.* 1st rev ed. New York, NY: Crown Publishers; 2005

Gabriels RL, Hill DE. *Autism: From Research to Individualized Practice.* London, England: Jessica Kingsley Publishers; 2002

Notbohm E. *Ten Things Every Child with Autism Wishes You Knew.* Arlington, TX: Future Horizons; 2005

Siegel B. *The World of the Autistic Child: Understanding and Treating Autism Spectrum Disorders.* New York, NY: Oxford University Press; 1996

Szatmari P. *A Mind Apart: Understanding Children With Autism and Asperger Syndrome.* New York, NY: Guilford Press; 2004

Wiseman ND, Koffsky KP. *Could It Be Autism? A Parent's Guide to the First Signs and Next Steps.* New York, NY: Broadway Books; 2006

Behavior Management, Social Skills, and Health

Bondy A, Frost L. *A Picture's Worth: PECS and Other Visual Communication Strategies in Autism*. 2nd ed. Bethesda, MD: Woodbine House; 2011

Durand VM. *Sleep Better! A Guide to Improving Sleep for Children with Special Needs*. Baltimore, MD: Paul H. Brookes Publishing Co; 1998

Ernsperger L, Stegen-Hanson T. *Just Take a Bite: Easy, Effective Answers to Food Aversions and Eating Challenges*. Arlington, TX: Future Horizons, Inc; 2004

Gray C. *The New Social Story Book*. 10th anniv rev ed. Arlington, TX: Future Horizons; 2010

Harris SL, Weiss MJ. *Right From the Start: Behavioral Intervention for Young Children With Autism*. 2nd ed. Bethesda, MD: Woodbine House; 2007

Howlin P, Baron-Cohen S, Hadwin J. *Teaching Children with Autism to Mind-Read: A Practical Guide for Teachers and Parents*. Chichester, England: J. Wiley and Sons; 1999

Kemper KJ. *Mental Health, Naturally: The Family Guide to Holistic Care for a Healthy Mind and Body*. Elk Grove Village, IL: American Academy of Pediatrics; 2010

Kluth P, Shouse J. *The Autism Checklist: A Practical Reference for Parents and Teachers*. San Francisco, CA: Jossey-Bass; 2009

Legge B. *Can't Eat, Won't Eat: Dietary Difficulties and Autistic Spectrum Disorders*. London, England: Jessica Kingsley Publishers; 2002

McClannahan LE, Krantz PJ. *Activity Schedules for Children with Autism: Teaching Independent Behavior*. 2nd ed. Bethesda, MD: Woodbine House; 2010

Moor J. *Playing, Laughing, and Learning with Children on the Autism Spectrum: A Practical Resource of Play Ideas for Parents and Careers*. 2nd ed. London, England: Jessica Kingsley Publishers; 2008

Myles BS, Southwick J. *Asperger Syndrome and Difficult Moments: Practical Solutions for Tantrums, Rage, and Meltdowns*. 2nd ed rev. Shawnee Mission, KS: Autism Asperger Pub; 2005

Naseef RA. *Special Children, Challenged Parents: The Struggles and Rewards of Raising a Child with a Disability.* Rev ed. Baltimore, MD: Paul H. Brookes Publishing Co; 2001

Notbohm E, Zysk V. *1001 Great Ideas for Teaching and Raising Children with Autism or Asperger's.* 2nd ed rev. Arlington, TX: Future Horizons; 2010.

Ozonoff S, Dawson G, McPartland J. *A Parent's Guide to Asperger Syndrome and High Functioning Autism: How to Meet the Challenges and Help Your Child Thrive.* New York, NY: Guilford Press; 2002

Schopler E. *Parent Survival Manual: A Guide to Crisis Resolution in Autism and Related Developmental Disorders.* New York, NY: Plenum Press; 1995

Siegel B. *Helping Children With Autism Learn: Treatment Approaches for Parents and Professionals.* New York, NY: Oxford University Press; 2003

Volkmar FR, Wiesner LA. *Healthcare for Children on the Autism Spectrum: A Guide to Medical, Nutritional and Behavioral Issues.* Bethesda, MD: Woodbine House; 2004

Wetherby AM, Prizant BM. *Autism Spectrum Disorders: A Transactional Developmental Perspective.* Baltimore, MD: Paul H. Brookes Publishing Co; 2000

Wheeler M. *Toilet Training for Individuals with Autism or Other Developmental Issues: A Comprehensive Guide for Parents & Teachers.* 2nd ed. Arlington, TX: Future Horizons; 2007

Wilens TE. *Straight Talk about Psychiatric Medications for Kids.* 3rd ed. New York, NY: Guilford Press; 2009

Adolescence and Adulthood

Baker J. *Preparing for Life: The Complete Guide for Transitioning to Adulthood for those with Autism and Asperger's Syndrome.* Arlington, TX: Future Horizons; 2005

Glasberg BA. *Functional Behavior Assessment for People with Autism: Making Sense of Seemingly Senseless Behavior.* Bethesda, MD: Woodbine House; 2006

Sicile-Kira C. *Adolescents on the Autism Spectrum: A Parent's Guide to the Cognitive, Social, Physical, and Transition Needs of Teenagers with Autism Spectrum Disorders.* New York, NY: A Perigee Book; 2006

Wrobel M, Rielly P. *Taking Care of Myself: A Hygiene, Puberty and Personal Curriculum for Young People with Autism.* Arlington, TX: Future Horizons; 2003

Magazines and Newsletters

Autism Asperger's Digest
336/222-0442

www.autismdigest.com

Magazine with current research, practical tips, and informative discussions on topics of concern to families with children and adults on the spectrum

The Autism File
www.autismfile.com

Quarterly magazine and Web site providing practical information about myriad aspects of autism, including treatments, nutrition, and education

Autism Spectrum News
508/877-0970

www.mhnews-autism.org

Quarterly publication that provides news, information, and resources about scientific research, evidence-based clinical treatments, and family issues

HOPELights
888/503-7553

www.hopelightmedia.com

Monthly activity magazine for children who have special needs, including autism

Appendix B
Early Intervention Program Referral Form

Please complete this form for referring a child to Early Intervention (Part C) if you prefer to do so in writing. Also please indicate the feedback that you want to receive from the Early Intervention Program in response to your referral. Diagnosis of a specific condition or disorder is not necessary for a referral.

Parent/Child Contact Information

Child Name: _____

Date of Birth: _____/_____/_____   Child Age: (Months) _____   Gender: M F

Home Address: _____

Parent/Guardian_____ Relationship to Child: _____

Primary Language: _____ Home Phone: _____ _____ Other Phone:_____

Reason(s) for Referral to Early Intervention

(Please check all that apply)

☐ Identified condition or diagnosis (e.g., spina bifida, Down syndrome): _____

☐ Suspected developmental delay or concern (Please circle areas of concern):

Motor/Physical   Cognitive   Social/Emotional   Speech/Language   Behavior   Other_____

☐ At Risk (Describe risk factors): _____

☐ Other (Describe): _____

Referral Source Contact Information

Person Making Referral: _____ Date of Referral: _____/_____/_____

Address: _____

Office Phone_____Office Fax: _____ E-mail_____

Early Intervention Program Contact Information

Program Name: _____

Address: _____City: _____ State: _____ Zip: _____

Office Phone_____Office Fax: _____ E-mail_____

Feedback Requested by the Referral Source

Date Referral Received: _____/_____/_____   Date of Initial Appointment with Child/Family: _____/_____/_____

Name of Assigned Service Coordinator: _____

Office Phone: _____ Office Fax: _____ E-mail: _____

After initial appointment, please send the following information:

☐ Status of Initial Family Contact   ☐ Changes in Services Being Provided

☐ Developmental Evaluation Results   ☐ Periodic Progress Reports/Summaries

☐ Services Being Provided to Child/Family   ☐ Other (Describe): _____
(Including: names of providers and frequency of services)   _____

Release of Information Consent

I,_____(Print name of parent or guardian), give my permission for my pediatric health care

provider, _____(print provider's name), to share any and all pertinent information regarding

my child,_____(print child's name), with the early intervention program.

Parent/Legal Guardian Signature_____ Date:_____/_____/_____

This form is available on the National Center of Medical Home Initiatives for Children with Special Needs website. Go to http://www.medicalhomeinfo.org/health/EI.html to download this form and learn more about Early Intervention.

This form was developed as part of a collaboration between the American Academy of Pediatrics and the Tracking, Referral and Assessment Center for Excellence, Orelena Hawks Puckett Institute, Inc. The development of this form was supported, in part, by funding from the US Department of Education, Office of Special Education Programs, Research to Practice Division (H324G020002).

Appendix C

Emergency Information Form for Children With Autism Spectrum Disorders

Today's date	
Your name	
Do you CONSENT to the release of this form to health care professionals?	◉ Yes ○ No
Is this a new form or an update?	

Information About the Child

Child's name		Primary address	
Birth date		City, state, zip	
Patient's nickname		Primary language	
Primary means of communication		Does he/she wear a medical ID bracelet?	
Parent/guardian #1		Parent/guardian #2	
Phone number		Phone number	
Emergency contact		Emergency contact	

Providers & Facilities

Care Provider	Provider's Name	Specialties	Office Number, Fax, and E-mail
Primary care			
Specialist 1			
Specialist 2			
Specialist 3			
Specialist 4			
Specialist 5			
Others			
Primary pharmacy (branch, phone, other)			
Anticipated primary emergency department (name, phone, other)			
Anticipated tertiary care center (name, phone, other)			

Clinical Information/Management Data

Diagnoses/past procedures (list all), starting with most important		1
		2
		3
		4
Baseline physical findings		
Baseline vital signs		
Most recent height and weight (including date)		
Baseline neurologic status		
Description of cognitive/developmental age for		
	Receptive language	
	Expressive language	
Description of cognitive skills		
Description of gross motor skills		
Description of fine motor skills		
Comfort items		
Does he/she wander off? If so, to where? Describe.		

Medications	Significant Laboratory Results (eg, blood tests, x-ray, ECG)
1	1
2	2
3	Technology Devices (eg, communication aids)
4	1
5	2

Allergies: Medications/Food to Be Avoided & Why	Procedures to Be Avoided & Why
1	1
2	2
3	3
4	4

Immunizations (mo/y)			
DPT dates		Varicella status	
DTaP dates		Hep B dates	
OPV or IPV dates		Hep A dates	
MMR dates		Meningococcal	specify which one if possible
Hib dates		TB status	
Pneumococcal-7		HP virus	
Pneumococcal-13		Influenza	
Rotavirus		Tdap	
Other		Other	

Comments on child, family, or other specific medical issues	

Physician/Provider Signature	Printed Name

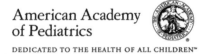

American Academy
of Pediatrics

DEDICATED TO THE HEALTH OF ALL CHILDREN™

Appendix D

Medication Flow Sheet

MEDICATION	DATE STARTED/ TARGET SYMPTOM(S)	DOSE CHANGES/ BENEFITS/SIDE EFFECTS	DATE DISCONTINUED, REASON
PATIENT:			

Adapted with permission from Alan Rosenblatt, MD, SC

Index